Where Will I Sleep?

A journey with childhood cancer from
diagnosis and treatment to lessons in faith

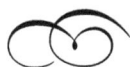

Rhonda Kay Diliberti

PARKVIEW PRESS

Copyright © 2012 by Rhonda Kay Diliberti.

Published by Parkview Publishing
Please send inquiries to: 55527 Parkview,
Shelby Township, MI 48316

First Edition: December 2012

Book Cover by Karrie Ross
Edited by Jane Denys-Myers

Library of Congress Cataloging-in-Publication Data
Where Will I Sleep?: A journey with childhood cancer from diagnosis
and treatment to lessons in faith / Rhonda K. Diliberti

ISBN: 978-0-615-43491-9

Printed in the United States of America.

HARDCOVER EDITION

This book is dedicated to Melissa and Elizabeth
who lived through the journey but were
perhaps too young to remember the details.
It is for you that this book is written.

Contents

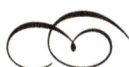

Acknowledgments

Jonathan's story has become a part of me. I know now that writing this book was a necessary part of my healing. It was also important to me to preserve Jonathan's memory and to share his gift of faith, for perhaps that was his true purpose in life. For these reasons, I am grateful to many who helped bring this book to completion. I would especially like to acknowledge the following individuals for their continued help, guidance, and support.

For creating the perfect backdrop from which to write each summer, I thank the entire Diliberti family. Your love, warmth, and expression of family is truly admirable.

To my mother, Mary Kay Eschenburg, who longed for this book as much as I did. Thank you for the editing remarks, chapter titles, and ever-present support.

To my late father, William Eschenburg, thank you for inspiring me to always work harder, reach higher, and strive for more. When this project seemed daunting, I always thought of you.

For knowing that I can count on them for anything, I thank my brother, Michael, and sister, Laurie. From trips to New York, to technical support, to always remembering Buzz, you both exemplify the true meaning of family.

To Jane Denys-Myers, thank you for editing the final manuscript. I am extremely grateful for your thoughtful comments and kind suggestions.

To Karrie Ross, thank you for the perfect cover. The soft snowy scene reminds me of the view outside my window and of the warmth we experienced during Jonathan's finals days.

For helping with the interior layout and for offering your design services many times throughout the years, I thank Laura Carruthers.

To Joann Eschenburg, thank you for your excitement about reading the first proof and for catching a number of errors.

For serving as my sounding board and crying with me, I thank my daughters, Melissa and Elizabeth Diliberti. Thank you, Melissa, for your many lessons on grammar and the use of commas. I'm not sure I passed, but I know this book is greatly improved after your many hours of work. To Elizabeth, thank you for serving as my assistant and for making the final decisions regarding the layout of this book. As always, your attention to detail is outstanding. I hope you both feel this book is equally yours.

To Thomas Diliberti, thank you for believing in me. Your support and encouragement throughout the years is what made this book happen. The love that transcends the pages of this book is also a tribute to you, for you are a wonderful husband and father. Thank you for allowing me to spend countless hours putting our story into book form.

And to all of you so deeply touched by Jonathan's message, thank you for encouraging me to write this book.

Foreword

When our 22-month-old son was first diagnosed with cancer, we were overwhelmed. Overwhelmed with how our lives had changed overnight, overwhelmed with the thought that our child might die, and even overwhelmed with the gracious outpouring of love and support that we received from others. After three days of the phone ringing incessantly with offers of help, I didn't want to talk to anyone except another mother whose child had cancer. Although the doctors could answer our medical questions, only another mom could tell me what to expect and how this shocking news was going to affect our lives. When Jonathan's cancer returned after an 8-month remission, we were once again devastated and in desperate need of hope and guidance. We began an exhaustive search for new information. While we found a lot of cancer facts, we found little information on living with cancer, what to expect, and even less on the kinds of decisions that we would eventually have to face.

For these reasons, I decided to chronicle our day-to-day trials and tribulations in an online journal. The daily updates allowed friends and family to keep abreast of Jonathan's treatment and progress, and I realize now that the act of journaling proved therapeutic for me. Unbeknownst to me at the start, the journal evolved into so much more as Jonathan lived his final months. Over the years, many people have encouraged me to put Jonathan's story into book form. While many of the entries in this book were originally part of the online journal, I have since gone back, filled in the holes, and reflected on our journey. This book details the complete story of our walk with cancer, from Jonathan's initial diagnosis to his everlasting gift.

I hope that reading about our journey will give newly diagnosed families some insight into living with cancer, for it was this type of information that I so desperately craved. I truly believe that knowledge can provide both strength and support. Our story may also provide friends and family some understanding of the cancer world and give some tangible clues as to how they can best help. This book may also give health professionals another perspective from which to view a childhood cancer family and perhaps serve as a loving reminder of the significance and value of their everyday work. Most importantly, I hope that Jonathan's spirit will cause you to remember the joy in everyday life and that you will discover for yourself Jonathan's gift.

In his four short years, Jonathan was able to inspire others more than most will do in a lifetime. He will remain in our hearts forever.

Rhonda
~ Mom to Melissa, Elizabeth, and Jonathan forever ...

A Word of Caution!

Without hope, you are not truly living.

Yes, you guessed it. My child died. But that does not mean that yours will too! If there is one thing I have learned about cancer, it is that we do not know nearly enough. I was initially frustrated with Jonathan's doctors because they could not provide for me a clear plan – a clear, detailed plan that you could project on the wall that would flowchart the path to curing my child. It actually took me a few months to understand that their lack of a plan was not a professional flaw but really a limitation of medical science and understanding.

Throughout our travels, we met a number of children with cancer. I can name children who had considerable disease, some worse than Jonathan, who are alive and well today. I can name others who had the same type of cancer with similar circumstances who responded very differently to the same treatment. We had the privilege of speaking with some of the best cancer researchers in the world. I was humbled by their passion and commitment to finding a cure for all children with cancer. Every day their efforts and research bring new hope and treatment possibilities. You must embrace this hope, for without it, you will not truly be living. Yes, my child died. But that does not mean that yours will too.

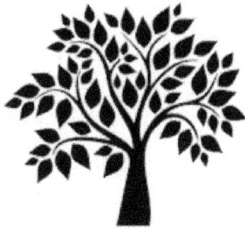

Meet the Family

Tom and I both come from very close families. I am the oldest of three children. My brother, Michael, lives in Washington, D.C. and is unmarried. My sister, Laurie, married Tom's best friend, Chris, two years after we married. Their two boys, Andrew and Matthew, were born soon after. My parents, William & Mary Kay Eschenburg, were affectionately named Grandma and Grandpa E by the grandkids. My Aunt Joann is also very much part of the immediate family.

In similar fashion, the grandchildren called Tom's parents, Tom and Mary Diliberti, Grandma and Grandpa D. Tom is the third of four children. His oldest sister, Lynn, married Sal a month after our wedding. They had Anna soon after. Tom's sister, Laura, married Tim a month later, and soon had Zachary. Their twins, Jessica and Samantha, were then born a few months after Jonathan. Tom's younger brother Dan is not yet married. We are generally one, big, happy family.

PART ONE

Meet Buzz

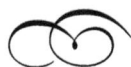

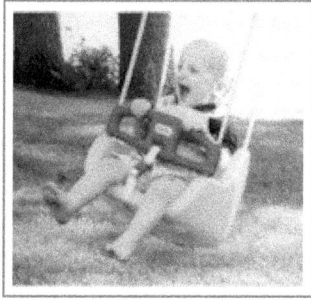

Introducing Buzz!

We had not planned on having another child, but … well, things happen. Jonathan Thomas Diliberti was born on April 28, 1996. Melissa was five. Elizabeth was three. While still in the hospital, the girls gave Jonathan his very first present: a soft, fuzzy, light blue baby blanket wrapped in a large box with ribbons going every which way with many, many bows. From that day on, his blanket was always nearby.

Jonathan was a very easy baby and, as a third child, he quickly melded into the family. He spent most of his time playing with his sisters and doing silly things to make everyone laugh. The extended family teased that he was loud and always making noise – from screaming and crying to constantly chattering. He did not like to sleep alone and climbed in most nights with his blanket between Mom and Dad.

We were a typical, busy, suburban family. Tom and I were both high school teachers. We had three children, a new house, a full-time babysitter, after-school activities, family and friends, and not enough time each day to accomplish all that needed to be done. But we were extremely content, and Jonathan was our happy child. With his perfectly round head and lack of hair, somewhere along the way we started calling him Buzz, as in Buzz Lightyear from Disney's Toy Story. Buzz was our reminder that some accidents have happy endings.

Life Takes a Turn

One Sunday morning, March 1st, 1998, to be exact, I noticed a small lump on Jonathan's head while washing his hair. It was soft to the touch, about an inch-and-a-half in diameter, but it didn't seem to bother him. Although we were not deeply concerned, we decided to take Jonathan to the weekend clinic rather than risk missing a day of work for a trip to the pediatrician later in the week. Tom took Jonathan to the walk-in clinic that evening while I got the girls ready for bed. The doctor on duty noted the lump on Jonathan's head and also felt something in his abdomen. He did some blood work and highly recommended that we take Jonathan to his pediatrician the following day. Even so, we were not particularly worried or alarmed. The next day our pediatrician also noted the lumps and immediately sent us to St. John Hospital for a number of tests.

The week quickly became a blur, one test after another, for days in a row—more blood work, a CAT scan, bone scan, x-rays, urine test, etc. Jonathan was terrified of the pokes and afraid of the many strangers invading his space. Clinging to his blanket, he generally sat on our laps and buried his face. It wasn't much better for us. One night was particularly heart-wrenching as we had to help hold Jonathan down while the medical team worked to insert a tube into his stomach through his nose. Kicking and screaming, Jonathan looked bewildered to see that his parents were actually partaking in the event. My most vivid memory, however, was the horror-stricken look on the lab technician's face when we asked her what the big, bright yellow spot was on the scan she had just completed. She quickly fumbled that we would have to wait until morning to discuss the results of the scan with the doctor. I was absolutely furious. How could she know something about our child and not tell us? I told her, in a not-so-pleasant voice, that we weren't going home until somebody told us what was going on. But it was 9:00 pm, and the place was dark and empty. So we had no choice. We went home, now worried, yet even more furious.

When we returned the next morning, Friday, March 6th, we were sent to an office. While waiting, I read the names on the door – Dr. Sawaf and Dr. Lorenzana, Oncologists. I quickly leaned over and asked Tom if he knew what "oncology" meant. Although it is somewhat embarrassing to admit now, the truth is that neither one of us knew the meaning of the word. We still had no idea what was wrong with our child.

Soon, we received our answer. After five days of tests and very little communication throughout the week, Jonathan, at age 22 months, was diagnosed with cancer – stage IV neuroblastoma. After Dr. Sawaf spelled neuroblastoma for me, he explained that a large tumor was found on Jonathan's adrenal gland and that the disease had already spread to his head and bone marrow. He then gently suggested we go home and try to enjoy the weekend because starting Monday, we would be entering a whole new world.

A Whole New World

The weekend, however, was far from enjoyable. Word of Jonathan's diagnosis spread very fast. Friends, relatives, and neighbors phoned when they first heard the news, and extended family gathered at our home. We spent most of the day on Saturday answering the phone, telling the same story over and over. In between, we searched the internet trying to learn as much as we could about cancer, neuroblastoma, treatment, prognoses, and what this all meant. The more we read, however, the worse we felt. By the end of the day, I could not look at Jonathan without starting to cry.

With a house full of people and the phone still ringing, I asked my mother to handle the incoming calls. I just couldn't talk anymore. The only person I wanted to talk to at that moment was another mother whose child had neuroblastoma. I had so many questions that did not have a "medical" answer, so many fears of what was to come. Unbelievably, Mary, one of our neighbors, who is also a dear friend, located a family nearby who had such a child. She gave me her number, and I phoned the mother out of the blue. The mother was more than willing to speak with me, and best of all, she completely understood all that I was feeling. We compared notes and details, and talked about what it was going to be like caring for a child with cancer. Secretly, I was most relieved when she said that her child no longer had neuroblastoma, and that their lives were back to normal. In the end, she reassured me that life would go on and that, in time, we would learn to adjust to this whole new world. Still shocked, but slowly accepting the impending reality, I stayed up most of the night reading all I could about cancer, neuroblastoma, and various cancer treatments. By Monday morning, we understood the facts and knew we faced a great battle.

Neuroblastoma

According to the American Cancer Society, cancer is a group of diseases characterized by the uncontrolled growth and spread of abnormal cells. Normal cells grow, divide, and die in an orderly fashion. Cancer occurs when a cell's DNA becomes damaged, and the cells begin to divide uncontrollably. As the cells continue to divide, they eventually form a visible mass or tumor. The cancerous cells can then spread to other parts of the body where they start new growths and cause further destruction. The type of cancer is determined by the organ in which the cancer originates and/or the kind of cell from which it is derived.

Neuroblastoma originates in the immature nerve cells of the sympathetic nervous system. Normally, these immature cells, called neuroblasts, differentiate and turn into mature nerve cells. Neuroblastoma results when the neuroblasts fail to mature and, instead, continue to grow and divide. Because clusters of these cells are normally found along the spine, in the abdomen, and in the adrenal glands, neuroblastoma most often originates in these locations. Although the actual cause of neuroblastoma is unknown, many scientists believe that the disease is caused by random mutations that occur during cell division rather than environmental factors.

Neuroblastoma is relatively rare, accounting for just 5% of all childhood cancers. That said, neuroblastoma affects approximately 1 in 100,000 children per year and is the third most common type of cancer in children. Ninety percent of all cases are diagnosed by the age of five. On rare occasions, the disease has been detected by ultrasound before birth and has been found in adults as well. Neuroblastoma is an aggressive cancer, and, in the majority of cases, the disease has already spread to other areas of the body at the time of diagnosis.

We also learned that cancers are identified by stage. The stage of a cancer is a general description of how far the cancer has spread in the body. In general, stage I cancers are confined to the original, primary site. These types of cancers are often operable and curable. Stage II and III cancers remain localized yet are more advanced and/or have started to spread. Stage IV cancers have already spread to other organs or parts of the body, and are, therefore, much more difficult to treat. While these are general descriptions, each stage is precisely defined for each type of cancer.

Jonathan's Case

Jonathan's case was classic. The abnormality felt in his abdomen by the clinic doctor and his pediatrician was a cancerous mass on his adrenal gland. The lump we felt on his head was a secondary growth due to the spreading of this original tumor. A bone marrow aspiration also detected numerous cancer cells throughout his bone marrow. Many children with such widespread disease start to limp or complain of body aches. Jonathan didn't seem to have any symptoms other than the visible lump on his head and the hidden mass in his abdomen.

Most importantly, we learned that the prognosis of long-term survival for a child with neuroblastoma depends on the age of the child, the stage of the disease, and biological markers characteristic of the disease. Neuroblastomas have been shown to spontaneously regress in infants under the age of one. Stage I cancers are generally more treatable than Stage IV cancers. And in neuroblastoma, some tumor markers are more favorable than others. Jonathan was over the age of one, had stage IV disease, and had "unfavorable" microscopic disease structure. The more we learned, the more it seemed that everything was stacked against us. In Jonathan's case, the statistics revealed less than a 10% chance of long-term survival.

What Do We Do?

With such poor odds, we questioned who to trust and where to go for treatment. We were scheduled to start treatment at St. John Hospital in Detroit. The initial tests were conducted at this hospital only because our pediatrician was affiliated with this facility. St. John Hospital is a local, community-based hospital forty-five minutes from our home. Children's Hospital of Michigan, also in Detroit, was about the same distance, and Mott Children's Hospital, affiliated with the University of Michigan, was an hour-and-a-half away. When we expressed hesitation about where to go for treatment, Dr. Sawaf kindly helped us secure a consultation with Dr. Abella, an oncologist at Children's Hospital of Michigan. Dr. Abella explained in great detail the various modes of cancer treatment and the "scientific method" of clinical trial research.

Scientists are trying to stop the spread of cancer in a variety of ways. Chemotherapy utilizes drugs to kill cancer cells. These chemicals target fast growing cells. So while these drugs may kill cancer cells, they also damage other fast-growing cells like hair and blood cells as well. Immunotherapies are designed to utilize one's own immune system to help destroy cancer cells. Other therapies are constructed to target specific stages of the cell cycle. Regardless of the modality, the goal of treatment is to stop the cancer cells from replicating, thus ending the cancer.

Dr. Abella went on to explain that scientists use carefully controlled research studies called clinical trials to test treatment protocols. Phase I trials are generally designed to evaluate the safety and appropriate dosage of first-time treatment therapies on humans. Successful therapies then progress to Phase II. Phase II clinical trials evaluate the effectiveness and side effects of the proposed therapy. Phase III clinical trials then compare the effectiveness of new treatment protocol to the current, best-effective, standard treatment therapy. As scientists continue to learn more, standard treatment therapies are continually compared, modified, and improved.

From a scientific standpoint, the path ahead was becoming clear. Because science did not have the answers we were looking for, we were now entering the field of true medical research. Standard treatment for stage IV neuroblastoma, at this time, involved high-dose chemotherapy, followed by surgery, radiation, and a bone marrow transplant. We learned that Jonathan's initial treatment protocol would, for the most part, be the same regardless of where he was treated. Because of this and for reasons of family convenience, we chose to stay at St. John Hospital.

Initial Treatment Protocol

Jonathan was initially treated according to the POG-93404 high-risk neuroblastoma protocol, a Phase III clinical trial. The chemotherapy regimen consisted of high dose cisplatin, cyclophosphamide, alternating with cyclophos-

phamide doxorubicin, vincristine, carboplatin, and ifos-
famide on a three-week schedule. Potential side effects were
numerous and long-lasting such as hearing loss, infertility,
developmental issues, and the risk of secondary cancers.
Jonathan had a tube called a Broviac catheter surgically
inserted into his bloodstream through his chest to provide
easy access for blood draws and chemotherapy. The hope
was that the chemotherapy would reduce the bulky disease,
and the residual treatment would get rid of any remaining
cancer cells.

Jonathan ultimately completed six rounds of chemotherapy. In general, he tolerated it well and accepted the hospital
routines. With the help of preventive medications, he
experienced minor nausea and vomiting. We often had to
return to the hospital post-treatment, however, to receive
blood transfusions and/or antibiotics for an infection.
When it was time to return to the hospital, Jonathan liked
to pack his own bag—more stuffed animals than we could
carry, a big box of toys, "vee-vee" (what he called his light
blue baby blanket), and lots and lots of oversized t-shirts
that he called "sleep shirts." Every time we were admitted
to the hospital, the nurse would gently lay a small hospital
gown and mask at the end of the bed for Jonathan. As soon
as the nurse left, Jonathan would push them away and
quickly put on one of his sleep shirts. He never did wear a
hospital gown or mask! And his blanket never left his side.
Vee-vee went through chemo, surgery, radiation, scans—you
name it. We would always warn the doctors that nothing
could happen to vee-vee. His light blue blanket was the one
and only. When Jonathan was a baby, we tried to introduce
a second light blue baby blanket into his world, so we could
more easily wash the first. We would tuck him in his crib
with a new, but identical blanket, and he would promptly

throw it out of his crib. After weeks of subtly trying to introduce the new blanket in a variety of ways, we gave up. It was obvious he recognized the imposter.

Jonathan lost his hair sometime after the second round of chemo, but it was barely noticeable as his hair had just recently started to grow. After the fourth cycle of chemotherapy, the adrenal tumor was surgically removed. The tumor measured 12 cm x 15 cm, which was extremely large for Jonathan's little body. Tom and I asked if we could see the tumor. While the request may seem odd to some, we are extremely grateful that his doctors were able to arrange this. After being led to the basement of the hospital, a pathologist showed us Jonathan's tumor. It was already in a jar with his name on it. We held it, poked it, and just stared at it. It was the size of a baked potato but felt soft like a plum. It was hard to believe that the lump of cells that we were holding was once inside our child and could be so devastating. So far, everything had been so surreal. Seeing the tumor helped me "visualize" the enemy.

Adjusting at Home

Undergoing treatment was a big adjustment for the entire family. When Jonathan was first diagnosed, Tom took an immediate leave of absence from his teaching position and put his graduate coursework on hold. I continued to teach to keep our medical benefits intact. Together, we tried hard to keep the girls' lives as stable as possible. Tom spent most of the nights in the hospital with Jonathan. Tom's parents or my parents would often relieve him in the morning and spend the day with Jonathan. I would come right after school and stay until Tom returned later that night. Tom usually had just enough time to go home, shower, mow the lawn, pay the bills, etc., before it was time to return. I would get up at 5:00 am, teach all day, spend the afternoon and evening at the hospital, put the girls to bed, and then stay up late doing lesson plans and researching cancer information into the wee hours of the morning. Our sitter, Donna, continued to get the girls off to school in the morning, and they usually spent the afternoon/evenings with friends or relatives. Sometimes Tom would bring the girls back to the hospital with him when he returned, and then they'd ride back home with me. Doing so allowed them to visit with Jonathan for a half-hour or so and gave me a chance to catch up with them on the drive home before tucking them in. At the hospital, Tom and I would share a quick hug, update each other as to what was happening, and then make the switch. We tag-teamed at the hospital and rarely had time to really talk to one another. Our lives were split between home and hospital – never knowing where we would be or how long we would be there. We missed being together. We missed being a family.

The initial chemotherapy regimen lasted five months. Jonathan completed this standard treatment protocol in July of 1998. With school out for summer, we finally had some quality family time. It felt so good to be home for an extended period of time. The kids played together, and even everyday chores felt glorious! We were even able to sneak in a three-day vacation to Kings Island with Lynn & Sal, and Tim & Laura, and all the kids. We all had a great time.

Jonathan's Bone Marrow Transplant

Within weeks, however, we began preparing for Jonathan's final treatment regimen – a bone marrow transplant. We knew that this was one of the most critical phases of his treatment. The goal of this part of the treatment was to receive an ultra-high dose of chemotherapy to eliminate any residual cancer cells that may have existed. High-dose chemotherapy, however, damages the bone marrow and, consequently, the stem cells from which new blood cells arise—hence, the need for a bone marrow or, more appropriately, a stem cell transplant.

Technically, Jonathan had an autologous, peripheral blood stem cell transplant (PBSCT). Autologous means that he received his own stem cells rather than getting them from someone else. Stem cells that leave the bone marrow and enter the bloodstream are called peripheral stem cells. In a PBSCT, stem cells are removed from the bloodstream and are then re-infused at a later date. The hope is that the re-infused stem cells make their way to the bone marrow and soon start producing healthy new blood cells.

Jonathan's stem cell transplant was guided by Dr. Abella, the same doctor we consulted with earlier, from Children's Hospital of Michigan. His stem cells were harvested the second week of August. We were then admitted to the Karmanos Cancer Center on August 26, 1998. Jonathan received one week of ultra high-dose chemotherapy and then had his actual transplant, in which his stem cells were re-infused, on September 2. The high-dose chemotherapy took a lot out of him. Jonathan had very little strength and no energy. Most of the people on the transplant floor were elderly adults. Jonathan was the anomaly. He was just a tiny lump in a big bed on the spacious floor. He spent most of his time sleeping. When he was awake, he watched Barney videos. We watched his favorite video, "Happy Birthday, Barney," over and over, and over again. And if we tried to turn the volume down, he would open one eye just wide enough to glare "turn that back up!" He also didn't have much of an appetite. When he did, he wanted pop and chicken nuggets – his normal diet of "healthy" foods. Luckily, there was a Wendy's in the basement corridor of the hospital complex. One day, when he was particularly determined to eat his chicken nuggets, he took a bite, threw up, took another bite, threw up, took another bite, threw up again and continued the routine with little regard to cause and effect. He eventually fell asleep holding the box of remaining nuggets.

The days at the Karmanos Center were particularly long and difficult. The hospital floor was uncomfortably quiet and sterile, and because most residents lacked an immune system, visitors were kept to an absolute minimum. The girls were not allowed to visit, and it was obvious that Jonathan greatly missed their presence. And Tom and I were tired – tired from months of hospitals stays and emotionally worn down by the uncertainty we faced each day. We are grateful for the nights my sister, Laurie, spent at the hospital, giving Tom and me a chance to reconnect and spend some quality time at home together with the girls. It was extremely difficult for all of us. But, little by little, Jonathan's blood counts started to recover. As his counts increased, he slowly regained his strength, energy, and personality. We spent twenty-six days at the Karmanos Center. Jonathan was released near the end of September. I can't even begin to describe how we felt the day he was discharged! Finally, back at home – together again as a family.

Thank You's

We survived these initial months of treatment with the help of many. Friends and family were a constant presence and often anticipated our daily needs even when we could

not. Our parents helped with the many hospital stays and
provided great emotional support for both us and the girls.
Our neighbors and co-workers coordinated meals and
delivered them to our home. Everyone helped with the girls
and assisted in their after-school activities. Their teachers
stopped by for visits and provided additional support at
school. And friends of friends offered tickets to events, sent
baskets and notes of support. And small gifts and piles of
cards arrived almost daily for Jonathan. Not only was the
help greatly appreciated, it also reminded us that we were
not alone. I don't know how we would have survived these
initial months on our own. We will always remember the
many, many genuine acts of kindness we witnessed and
received. I hope that we can do the same for others.

Post-Bone Marrow Transplant

Yes, we were home, but things were still far from normal.
With Jonathan's immune system still very weak, we were
advised to adhere to a long list of precautions for the first
100 days post-transplant. We washed our hands many times
a day, changed our clothes upon entering the house, bought
a new vacuum cleaner, bleached anything and everything,
kept visitors to a minimum, and made Jonathan stay
indoors. Except for a secret trip to McDonald's drive-
through so Jonathan could order his own chicken nuggets,
we stayed home and just enjoyed being together. Tom
returned to work in October as Jonathan was doing
extremely well. He was eating, gaining weight, and his blood
counts were continuing to increase. He had post-treatment
tests in mid-December, and, right after Christmas, we got
the best news ever. Jonathan's scans and biopsies showed
"no evidence of disease." In January of 1999, Jonathan was

declared in remission!

Fast forward to April 1999 ... At this time, Jonathan's doctors recommended radiation therapy to the tumor site on his head. They believed that this might help prevent a recurrence at this location and/or would irradiate any microscopic residual disease. Jonathan eased through two weeks of radiation therapy with no side effects other than the loss of hair near the site. He just looked like he got a bad haircut!

We had just recently attended the St. John Cancer Survivor's Day picnic and really thought we were one of the lucky few. Yet we were still very nervous about his post-treatment nine-month work-up. In June 1999, we spent a day at Children's Hospital of Michigan undergoing a variety of tests. The next week was extremely nerve-racking as the results trickled in little by little and nothing was conclusive by itself. Also, Tom had confided that he saw some glowing yellow spots on the MIBG scan so we were particularly anxious for a complete summary.

The Dreaded News

On Monday, June 21st, we learned that Jonathan's cancer was back. We knew that if a child relapsed, the odds for long-term survival dramatically decreased. Now what?? I frantically started reading journal articles on recurrent neuroblastoma. It was obvious that we were in uncharted territory. There was no right or wrong answer nor a clear path to follow. Understanding, but frustrated by the lack of information at this juncture, it was here that I decided to start chronicling our walk with cancer in an online journal. The subsequent entries come from the Journal.

PART TWO

Enduring Trials

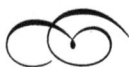

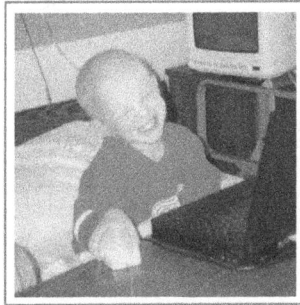

June/July 1999

Monday, 6/28 ~ Gathering research

Well, now that we know that Jonathan's cancer is back, I am back in research mode. My brother, Michael, came home from Washington, D.C. to lend his emotional and technical support. He re-configured my computer and helped me subscribe to a great neuroblastoma email group through the Association of Cancer Online Resources (ACOR). The group consists of parents of children with neuroblastoma from around the world. Let's just say that these parents are not passive! With the help of this group, I quickly accumulated a list of the top neuroblastoma researchers and research institutions. I can't imagine being in this situation without the internet!

Tuesday, 7/6 ~ Investigating treatment options

Today we met with Dr. Abella at Children's Hospital. The results of Jonathan's most recent scans showed two new tumors on his skull bone—one above his right eye, the other on his forehead. The original site on his head, which had been radiated, also looked suspicious. Regardless, the disease is back and is most likely present microscopically throughout the body. Dr. Abella outlined four general treatment modalities: chemotherapy, radiotherapy, immunotherapy, and "do nothing." He estimated that "doing nothing" would give Jonathan 6-8 weeks to live. For the most part, the options discussed were Phase I or Phase II clinical trials. Because these patient studies are so new and often involve so few patients, the data we are looking at to help guide our decision-making process is extremely limited or, at times, even non-existent. Jonathan seems so normal and full of life that, at this point, Tom and I do not feel that "doing nothing" is an option. We are currently researching all possible clinical trials. We had family over this evening to share this news and information.

Wednesday, 7/7 ~ Getting recommendations

I spent the entire day today researching information. With the help of my email group, I obtained the phone numbers and email addresses of the neuroblastoma researchers who are conducting the actual clinical trials. I wrote a somewhat generic letter and emailed each of them to ask for advice and/or information. I was surprised and humbled to get a response back from most of them by the end of the day. Two of them even called me on the phone. It is obvious that they are deeply compassionate and understand that time is of the essence. Many are suggesting a chemotherapy regimen with topotecan and cytoxin. (This same treatment was also suggested by Dr. Abella yesterday.) This chemo regime is currently a Phase II protocol. The doctors say that we should expect some kind of response from these drugs but stress that this treatment will not be a cure by itself.

Their thought is that it might buy us time as we (and they) continue to search for better options. I also scheduled an appointment with Dr. Val Castle, a researcher from the University of Michigan, as I saw her name in a number of research articles. We also purchased a new video camera and scheduled a family portrait session.

Monday, 7/12 ~ Visited U-M Cancer Center

We visited Dr. Castle at Mott Children's Hospital in Ann Arbor today. We heard the same thing – "neuroblastoma at this point is very resistant to treatment." She echoed that researchers are currently testing many different methodologies to kill neuroblastoma cells, but gently stated that she does not predict a cure for this disease in her lifetime. She indicated that the treatment options for recurrent neuroblastoma at this time are yielding a 1-3% event-free survival rate. She also reminded us to remember that many of these studies are still pending and that the "results" of these studies are still very premature. She highly suggested that we look into the research taking place at Memorial Sloan-Kettering Cancer Center (MSKCC) in New York City.

Wednesday, 7/14 ~ Consultation

We met with Dr. Sawaf, Jonathan's primary oncologist at St. John Hospital, this afternoon. We shared with him what we learned so far and discussed the various treatment protocols we found on the international Clinical Trial Database. Dr. Sawaf helped us sort through the research articles and patiently answered our many questions. We are leaning toward using the topotecan/cytoxin protocol suggested by many of the researchers because the outcomes appear to be statistically similar to other treatment options and the chemo can be administered at our local hospital. After the chemo regime, however, we all agree that we must do something else. At this point, we have no clear plan or protocol for the future. We went to Cedar Point this evening with Lynn & Sal, Laurie & Chris, and all the kids. We had a lot of fun, and it was a much needed distraction.

Friday, 7/16 ~ Family portrait taken
We had a family portrait taken this afternoon. Jonathan's eye is still partially closed and slightly swollen, but we wanted to get a picture before he lost his hair. We were glad that our local portrait studio was able to squeeze us in.

Saturday, 7/17 ~ Surgery
Jonathan had a metaport inserted today. This port looks like a button and is placed under the skin. It provides easy access to his bloodstream and provides a lot more freedom than the Broviac "tubies" he had before. He can even swim with his port! Surgery went well, although he is a little sore.

Because clinical trials also have certain "requirements," we hope to meet with the doctors at Memorial Sloan-Kettering in New York to learn more about their research before starting the chemo regime. We know that if we make a wrong move, we may eliminate Jonathan from a potential, future study.

Sunday, 7/18 ~ Visited churches
I visited a number of churches today. Tom and I think that starting to attend church regularly might be helpful to our family. With a little advance planning, I was able to attend at least a portion of six services this morning. Still looking for the right one …

Someone from the Make-A-Wish Foundation phoned this morning. She said that they received our name, but needed to talk to Jonathan's doctor to make sure he "qualifies" for a wish. I wonder who gave them our name ...

Monday, 7/19 ~ Gathering medical records
I spent most of the day on the phone trying to gather miscellaneous information – dates, doctors, medical records, etc. Arrangements are in progress for going to New York. I plan to call tomorrow to schedule the actual appointment.

Tuesday, 7/20 ~ Coordinating with four hospitals!
Today was a very productive day. We scheduled a consultation visit with Jonathan's radiation oncologist, Dr. Chuba, at Harper Hospital for Thursday. We are investigating doing local radiation to the tumor above Jonathan's eye. Between the tumor and a bug bite, his eye was barely open today.

I was then on the phone back and forth between Dr. Sawaf at St. John Hospital in Detroit and Dr. Cheung from Memorial Sloan-Kettering in New York City trying to work out all the details of our trip and Jonathan's subsequent treatment. You can learn more about the research taking place at MSKCC at their website, www.mskcc.org. (Incidentally, Memorial Sloan-Kettering was recently rated #1 in the country by U.S. News and World Report for cancer care! That makes me feel a little bit better.)

Dr. Cheung was much more optimistic on the phone than the previous researchers we talked to. His protocol consists of ultra high-dose chemotherapy followed by "3F8 monoclonal antibodies." We can do the high-dose chemo here in Michigan but would have to travel back and forth to New

York City to receive the antibody treatment. Dr. Cheung's current clinical trial is based on some of his earlier research. (I found an abstract of his earlier research in the Journal of Clinical Oncology. My mother, a city librarian, is ordering the full-text article for us through the library exchange.) Dr. Cheung would like us to be in New York on Monday and Tuesday for tests and a consultation visit. We will most likely fly out Sunday evening and stay at the New York Ronald McDonald House.

We also still need to have two more tests done here before we go. Right now I am trying to schedule an MRI and PET scan at Children's Hospital of Michigan because St. John Hospital does not have a PET machine. When I called Children's to schedule the PET scan, they said "Sorry, we are booked for months!" We don't have months!! So now I'm going back and forth between St. John and Children's Hospital trying to find someone who can help me get a scan ASAP. No one seems to understand the urgency of my request! We are also waiting for the social worker at MSKCC to call back with final details of our visit.

Tom and I are also trying to schedule a short, get-away vacation with Tim & Laura and kids before we go.

Thursday, 7/22 ~ All set to go!
I have been on the phone off and on all day for the past three days! We have finally ironed out all details. We are leaving this evening to go up north to Traverse City with Tim & Laura. We plan to return late Saturday night and have a flight into LaGuardia on Sunday morning. Jonathan is scheduled for a bone marrow biopsy and aspiration on Monday morning, and we will meet with Dr. Cheung in the

afternoon. We have a return flight on Tuesday. Jonathan is looking forward to riding in Uncle Tim's boat while Up North and flying in an airplane – all within days!

We got the PET scan done this morning at Detroit Children's Hospital and met with Dr. Chuba, a radiologist at Harper Hospital, to talk about Jonathan's eye. Both Dr. Cheung and Dr. Chuba think the chemotherapy may shrink the tumor above Jonathan's eye. For this reason, we have decided to wait on radiating at this time.

We have secured copies of all of Jonathan's medical records and have completed all the necessary scans. We are looking forward to hearing what the doctors at MSKCC recommend for our next phase of treatment. I am realistically optimistic. I will post again when we return.

7/22–7/24 ~ Up North having fun!

7/25–7/27 ~ In New York and I don't like it

Thursday, 7/29 ~ Back home
Wow, it has been a busy, crazy week. We had a great time at Tim's parents' cottage on Lake Ann near Traverse City. We enjoyed swimming, boating, playing, and just hanging out. Jonathan even went tubing with Daddy! We returned home, did a few midnight loads of laundry, and left for New York the following morning. I don't know if it was nerves or motion sickness, but I threw up during most of the flight. Dramamine saved me on the flight home. We stayed at the Ronald McDonald House, spent most of our time at the hospital, and returned home to spoiled food in the refrigerator because we had lost power. We had one

day to recover, then returned to St. John Hospital today.

We also received word that Jonathan qualified for "Make-A-Wish." Is that good news or bad news??

The trip to MSKCC was both informative and disappointing. It was confirmed that Jonathan does not have great odds. Memorial Sloan-Kettering, however, seems to be the "neuroblastoma capital" of the world. The doctors and researchers at MSKCC treat more neuroblastoma patients than any other hospital in the world. In fact, there were a number of neuroblastoma families living at the Ronald McDonald House from various other countries. If they have the financial means, this seems to be the choice destination. I also met some of the parents that I have been corresponding with via the listserv. It was so nice to finally meet them and their children in person!

We are intrigued with the monoclonal antibody treatment. This is a targeted therapy that attempts to use one's own immune system to kill cancer cells. From what I gathered, the hypothesis is something like this: Our immune system makes antibodies to attack foreign substances. The human immune system, however, does not attack cancer cells because the cancer cells originate from cells in our body. An antibody called 3F8, originally produced by the white blood cells of mice, is modified for human use in the lab and then given intravenously to a patient. The 3F8 mouse antibodies then circulate in the bloodstream and eventually attach to a GD2 protein that is found on the surface of all neuroblastoma cells. The hope is that the human body will eventually produce an antibody against the foreign 3F8 mouse antibodies. This secondary antibody is called a

HAMA ~ human-anti-mouse-antibody. Successive rounds of 3F8 infusions are given over time until the patient acquires a HAMA.

Jonathan must be free of bulky disease, however, to begin this treatment. In addition to the three tumors on his head, we learned in New York that the disease has increased in his bone marrow since June, and that he has small spots in his abdomen, on his spine, and in his leg. All day yesterday, Tom and I again wrestled with the various treatment options – this time including not treating at all. On the advice of Jonathan's doctors, we decided to take it one day or one week at a time. That was helpful advice. We agreed to use MSKCC's protocol of very high dose chemotherapy (topotecan and cyclophosphamide) here at St. John Hospital in attempt to rid him of bulky disease. The MSKCC protocols use higher doses of chemotherapy than many others because, in general, the higher the dose, the greater the response. Increased dosages, however, bring greater risks and side effects. So yes, you can kill cancer cells with increased dosages, but at some point, you will most likely kill everything else as well. Like everyone, we are looking for that perfect dose.

Jonathan began receiving the high-dose chemo regimen today. It will run for three days. We all agreed that we needed to see how well he tolerated the chemotherapy and to look for signs of improvement before deciding on any next steps. One of the tumors is still causing his right eye to be partially closed. We will use this to gauge progress. If all goes well, he will begin a second round of high-dose chemo three weeks from now. The doctors will then re-scan and assess his progress at that time.

Right now, I'm at home with the girls, and Tom is spending the night with Jonathan in the hospital. I bet they're watching sports on TV as we speak. ..."Daddy, who do you want to win – the red team or the blue team?"

Sunday, 7/31 ~ Elizabeth's birthday!
Three days into chemo and Jonathan is doing great! He is playing with toys, working puzzles, and watching videos – just like at home. We celebrated Elizabeth's 6th birthday in the hospital this evening with Grandma and Grandpa D. The ice cream cake was a bit melted, but it was great to be together. Happy Birthday, Bit!!

August 1999

Week of 8/1 ~ Home from hospital
Jonathan finished his first round of chemo and, after four days in the hospital, was released this evening. Surprisingly, the chemo didn't seem to faze him. He spent his days flipping through books, setting up his train, working puzzles, watching Teletubbies, or playing with his many visitors – Grandma and Grandpa D, Grandma and Grandpa E, Aunt Laurie & Uncle Chris, Aunt Laura & Uncle Tim, and his two sisters! His favorite line was "What we gonna do now?" (Mommy and Daddy are tired!) After the nurse disconnected his IV, he ran down the hall and was playing baseball at twin cousins', Jessica and Samantha's, birthday party an hour later. So much for the concerns of high-dose chemo! The doctors expect his blood counts to drop by Thursday/Friday though and his hair to fall out within a few weeks.

Monday, 8/2 ~ Back to normal
Tom took Elizabeth and Jonathan to the Tigers game

tonight where they met up with the rest of the family—
grandpas, aunts, uncles, cousins, etc. Jonathan was sooo
excited. He took his mitt and ball, wore his Tigers hat, and
loudly sang "Take Me Out to the Ball Game" during the
seventh inning stretch. The kids also got to run the bases
after the game. It was touching that when Elizabeth noticed
Jonathan lagging behind, she went back to re-run the bases
with him. All seemed to have a great time! I stayed home
to do more research and to catch up on things around the
house.

Friday, 8/6 ~ Back to the hospital
Well, today is Friday. As expected, Jonathan's blood counts
have dropped drastically. His ANC (absolute neutrophil
count), a measure of the body's ability to fight infection,
was 5 this morning. Normal ANC's are about 2000-6000.
Anything less than 500 poses a severe risk of infection. So,
not surprisingly, by mid-afternoon, he was running a
fever—a sure sign that his body was trying to fight something. So we are back at the hospital. In the past, these types
of stays have ranged from 3-10 days. Being told that we had
to return to the hospital really didn't seem to bother
Jonathan, but he whimpered when he left, "Me don't want
no pokes!" He's had more than his fair share of pokes the
last few weeks!

Jonathan was not himself today. He complained that his
body hurt and he wanted to be held all day. I got him to
take some chewable Tylenol today. (He does not readily
accept "med!") I convinced him that the new bubble gum
flavored pills were vitamins. Vitamins are ok, med is not!
I'm worried about my baby ...

Sunday, 8/8 ~ Feeling better!

Jonathan seems to be feeling much better today. His temperature has been normal since this morning and his cultures are still negative. He got up, watched some videos, and then worked diligently to set up his battery-operated train on his bed. As soon as he finished his food tray arrived. And when the food tray arrives, the routine is always the same. Slowly put away all the toys. Straighten the bed. Clean off the table. Rearrange the room to move the table closer. Make sure all tubes and wires are out of the way. Then Jonathan would sit up like a king, neatly arrange the silverware, slowly remove the cover, look down at the food, and then go, "YUUUCKKKKKK" and slam the lid down—every time! Basically, if it wasn't a chicken nugget, he wasn't interested! He ate goldfish crackers instead and then popped in another video.

I have been spending the days with Jonathan and Tom has been spending the nights. Jonathan likes to see the girls when we trade places.

Tuesday, 8/10 ~ Blood transfusions

Jonathan will be receiving red blood cells this evening and platelets tomorrow morning. We hope to go home—fully fueled—after this.

Wednesday, 8/11 ~ Back home – finally!

So after five days in the hospital, Jonathan was released about noon today. His temperature has been normal for the past three days and his cultures are still negative. But because he doesn't have any white blood cells, he came home on IV antibiotics. A home care nurse came out this afternoon to show us how to attach and detach the antibiotic to his line. We run his antibiotic every eight hours. Jonathan has been tolerating everything very well except for his daily "poke." He receives a shot of neupogen every evening to help his white count recover. Daddy "nurse" handles this because Mommy can't! My job is to snug him while Tom gives the shot and then comfort him afterward. It's going to be hard keeping him indoors for the next few days when it is so nice outside. We relented this evening and brought in his ride-in, battery-operated car from the garage. We watched him do laps around the newly painted basement floor and leave black skid marks along the way. Oh, well. In the big scheme of life, these kinds of things just don't matter anymore. It feels good to be home and great to be a family again. Thanks to all who helped us get through this past week.

Thursday, 8/12 ~ Losing hair fast …

Jonathan's hair is falling out in clumps. We took a before and after shower picture. One more shower, and it will be gone! Mom is sad. The home care nurse has been coming every day for blood draws. His ANC is still zero. Dr. Sawaf clarified that Jonathan will stay on antibiotics until his ANC reaches 300, and he will continue receiving the daily neupogen shot until his ANC is greater than 500.

Sunday, 8/15 ~ Counts are rebounding

Jonathan's white blood cells are starting to increase. His ANC was 153 today. His platelets, however, have dropped to 27,000. (Normal range is between 150,000-450,000.) He is scheduled to begin round two of chemo on Wednesday. He cannot begin this next round, however, until his ANC is at least 500 and his platelets are greater than 100,000. He also still has a few stray hairs. Elizabeth helped wash his hair today and said "That didn't take long!" Losing his hair doesn't seem to bother him.

Tuesday, 8/17 ~ No more pokes!

Jonathan's ANC is 2008 today! No more daily pokes, and Dr. Sawaf said he can start resuming normal activities. Translation—Jonathan wants to go to McDonalds and Chuck-E-Cheese. His platelets, however, are only 18,000. It looks like round two of chemo won't start until Monday.

Monday, 8/23 ~ Back to school and hospital

My stress level is skyrocketing!! Jonathan was scheduled to begin his second round of chemo today. Being that today was my first day of school and that Tom doesn't start until next week, Tom took Jonathan to the hospital this morning. Tom called at noon and said that Jonathan's last urine test came back "abnormal." As a result, the second round of chemo was postponed and a creatinine test to assess kidney function was ordered. If Jonathan's kidney function has been compromised, Dr. Sawaf will confer with Dr. Cheung in New York to determine the maximum dose of chemotherapy they feel he can safely incur. The first abnormal urine test suggests that the chemo may have to be scaled back to about 25% of his last dosage. We should have the results of the creatinine test by tomorrow morning.

These decisions are so hard to make. Right now, Jonathan's only hope of survival depends on him receiving ultra high-dose chemotherapy—higher than what he received during his initial treatment being that some of the initial cancer cells survived. In doing so, however, we may actually decrease his lifespan and quality of life if his body cannot tolerate the treatment. We are trying to carefully walk the line, making one decision at a time based on the data we have, and pray for clear signs to guide us. It is even harder when he looks and acts like a normal two year old – running around, riding his bike, yelling, screaming, playing with Melissa and Elizabeth, so full of energy and so full of life!

Tuesday, 8/24 ~ Kidney test ok!

Great news: the kidney test came back normal! Jonathan resumed the high-dose chemo this afternoon. We should be back home by Friday evening. We celebrated my birthday at the hospital this evening. Thanks for the birthday cupcakes, Mary!

Wednesday, 8/25 ~ Buzz is still Buzz!

Jonathan was his normal self today. He humored everyone on the floor as he roamed the halls, naked except for his choo-choo underwear and the "tubies" hanging from his chest, saying "Hello" to everyone he passed. In between, he said, "Come on Momma, let's skip! Come on Momma, let's hop!!" After a full day at school, Mom just didn't have enough energy to hop and skip!! He also told the "doc" this morning that his food was bad!

Friday, 8/27 ~ Back at home

Jonathan finished his second round of chemo about 5:30 pm this afternoon. We were home by 7:00 pm. We hope to take advantage of normal counts this weekend and do something fun as a family. We then have to schedule follow-up scans. His doctors expect him to be back in a few days for antibiotics and/or transfusions … just like always.

Sunday, 8/29 ~ Back to school

Tom starts school tomorrow and the girls start on Tuesday.

I am hoping that Jonathan can make it through the week on an outpatient basis. I have been researching home and/or outpatient chemotherapy options. I spent the week-end gathering information from other parents on the neuroblastoma listserv. It seems that some hospitals offer such an option. St. John Hospital does not have a home or outpatient chemo program in place, and they don't seem particularly interested in starting one. (They don't seem to like many of my great ideas!) I just don't think it is necessary to spend as much time as we do in the hospital "monitoring" or running hydration, nor do I think it is in the best interest of Jonathan. Plus, being away from home takes its toll on the entire family. Why can't we go home each night, tuck the kids in, sleep in our own beds, and return early the next morning?? Especially at this stage of the game …

Tuesday, 8/31 ~ Girls' first day of school
Today was Melissa and Elizabeth's first day of school. Melissa started third grade, Elizabeth started first. I took the day off so I could join the other moms at the bus stop and at school. (Good thing, as the bus never came!) Jonathan spent the day at my sister, Laurie's, with a new sitter, as we are not yet sure of our child-care needs. We're on the way back to the hospital right now, though, as Jonathan needs a red blood cell transfusion.

September 1999

Thursday, 9/2 ~ Another fever
Jonathan and I got home from the hospital last night a little after midnight. I don't understand why a three-hour blood cell transfusion takes over eight hours to complete!! I lost my patience with the admitting nurse when she was, from

my perspective, wasting my precious quality family time asking standard admitting questions such as, "Does he have any allergies? Are there any drugs or alcohol in the home? Can you describe his birth??" Aghhhhhhh!!! Just look at last week's chart!!!!!!!! Luckily, it looks like last year's PowerPoint will work well for tomorrow's lesson at school.

But today was a new day, and I was trying to get over my frustration from last night. Things were going fairly well until dinner. Halfway through dinner, Jonathan ripped off his shirt and yelled, "I'm hot!" Yes, he had a fever – most likely due to low blood counts. After talking with Dr. Sawaf on the phone, we were advised to bring him in. It is 11:15 pm. Tom and Jonathan just left for the hospital. Now it's sub plans, a change in childcare arrangements, a fever, another hospital stay, and it's only the second week of school. I'm going crazy ...

Saturday, 9/4 ~ We're home ...
After being admitted over 24 hours, Jonathan was released this morning on antibiotics. Melissa and Elizabeth seemed to miss Mom, Dad, and Buzz more than usual this week. I'm sad that we weren't around much for their first week of school. The girls and Melissa's best friend, Michelle, spent yesterday making pictures and "Get Well" cards for Buzz. They hung them on the front of the garage doors so that Jonathan would see them when he first got home. He noticed them right away and had me take a picture of him in front of the Teletubbies.

Monday, 9/6 ~ Overnight transfusions
Jonathan had his blood drawn at a local clinic yesterday. Soon after, Dr. Sawaf called and said he needed both red

blood cells and platelets. We decided to let these run overnight rather than lose a precious day at home. So Tom took Jonathan to the hospital last night about 9:30 pm. They returned home about 10:30 am this morning. We have another blood draw scheduled for tomorrow.

2nd post of the day: It is now evening and it looks like Jonathan's metaport site is infected. We just talked with Dr. Sawaf again. We agreed to do another round of antibiotics at home this evening and then pull the line. Jonathan will have to go back in tomorrow morning.

Tuesday, 9/7 ~ Back in the hospital

We don't really know what is going on at the moment. Jonathan's metaport site is red and inflamed; his skin is blotchy; he has purple dots on his head and face, and he said his body itches. This is not his normal response to chemo! But, as always, he is in good spirits. Mom had to go buy Cheez-Its, a Happy Meal, and Skittles. (He eats sooo healthy!) He did laps around the floor tonight, pointing to room after room as he passed. "Me was in that room!" ... "Me was in that room!" ... "Me was in that room!" ... etc. He was right; we've been in most all of them! His name and self-portrait is currently hanging on the wall in Pediatrics, and we were recently given an employee discount card to the hospital cafeteria. St. John Hospital—our new home away from home.

Wednesday, 9/8 ~ "Who gonna stay with me?"

Today, for the first time ever, we left Jonathan alone at the hospital for about two hours. I was so nervous and afraid!! Tom has spent most of the nights with Jonathan and said he was sure that Jonathan would not wake up before 9:00 am. I was so afraid of Jonathan waking up and discovering that he was all alone that I was reluctant to enact the plan. But if he slept until 9:00 am as usual, we had coverage for the day.

Tom spent the night at the hospital, got ready, and left for school at 6:00 am. Grandma and Grandpa E arrived about 8 am. Well, Tom was right! Grandma E. said Jonathan woke up about 9:15 am, rolled over, and said, "Hi, E!" He didn't seem to notice or remember that Daddy wasn't there anymore.

With the help of family and friends, Tom and I have been able to maintain our teaching schedules (and thus our jobs) when Jonathan is admitted to the hospital. I drop the girls off at Julie's (a neighbor and good friend down the street) in the morning, who gets them off to school. One of our parents stays with Jonathan during the day, while Tom and I are at school. I then go directly from school to the hospital, and Tom gets home in time to meet the girls' bus. The girls then spend the evening with family or neighbors while Tom returns to the hospital to spend the night. I try to head home as soon as possible, so I can chat with the girls before they fall asleep and iron out the details for the following day. It's getting to be somewhat of a routine. Tomorrow Daddy gets to spend his free time after school at the girls' dance studio!

Jonathan looks much better today, but his counts are still low. I need to catch one of the doctors tomorrow afternoon to get a better update on our situation. Not being here in the mornings means that we miss the doctors as they do their morning rounds. I returned home this evening to

18 voice messages and 129 emails! Needless to say, I'll get back to you … someday.

Thursday, 9/9 ~ Moment of truth …
Jonathan looked great today, and had lots of energy. He spent the day playing and running laps around the floor again. His counts are also increasing. Once his platelet count fully recovers, we will consider a third round of chemo. He also had a CAT scan today of his head, chest, and abdomen. The results of this scan (and next week's bone marrow aspiration) will guide our next course of treatment. We should have a preliminary report tomorrow. Please cross your fingers and send your prayers …

Tuesday, 9/14 ~ Scans look clear!!
We received the results of the CAT scan today. Great news: all the scans came back clear!! Jonathan's cancer seems to be responding well to the chemotherapy. He has now completed two rounds of chemo and has two more to go. We are scheduled to begin the third round using cisplatin and VP-16 on Thursday. This round should run through next Tuesday or Wednesday. A bone marrow aspiration will then take place next Thursday morning.

We also met with two representatives from the Make-A-Wish Foundation last night. They explained that the child has to articulate his or her wish to them directly without any assistance or coaxing from the family. To facilitate this request, we decided to meet them at our local Borders bookstore. We explained to Jonathan that two ladies were going to come to ask him some questions. When they arrived, Jonathan sat with them, as Tom and I sat a few tables away. Jonathan seemed relaxed as he answered their questions. When they asked him to describe his "wish," he said he wanted to "go to Disney World to meet Mickey Mouse in a hot air balloon." I am not really sure where he came up with that as we have never been to Disney, we don't have any Mickey Mouse paraphernalia, and we certainly haven't exposed him to hot air balloons!! We now have a lot of paperwork to complete to get the ball rolling, and we have to choose the best time to try to schedule the trip.

Thursday, 9/16 ~ Chemo postponed

I don't like these kinds of days! Nothing went as planned. I took the day off from school because Jonathan's chemo was scheduled to begin this morning. Because the kidneys have to be functioning at full capacity in order to tolerate the chemo drug, cisplatin, we submitted a urine sample a few days ago for a creatinine clearance test. Someone from the hospital phoned this morning to say that, for some unknown reason, the lab never completed the test. So the chemo was put on hold until the test could be completed. Dr. Sawaf then phoned a bit later to say that the lab just completed the test, but it appeared that Jonathan's kidneys were functioning well below average, just like before. So he wanted to perform a GFR test (another kidney test – supposedly more accurate.) This test came back normal but, after consulting with Dr. Cheung in NYC, it was decided to repeat the GFR test before administering the chemo. They said they just couldn't take a chance on poor kidneys. So now the plan is to complete the GFR test on Sunday and begin chemo on Monday. If the GFR test goes well, Jonathan will receive cisplatin; if not, we will repeat the cytoxin. While we were at the hospital, Jonathan did have a bone marrow aspiration (we should have results tomorrow) and an EKG (test results showed a great heart!!). While I am frustrated with the delay, I am so glad that we will be home for the weekend. I have to think of something fun to do …

Monday, 9/20 ~ Kidney is fine …

We enjoyed having a normal weekend – so much so that we chose not to do anything special. The GFR test came back normal, so we are scheduled to begin cisplatin this afternoon. It looks like Jonathan will be in the hospital through the weekend, and his doctors predict that this round will be his worst. We also learned from Dr. Lorenzana today that the chemo has greatly minimized the disease in Jonathan's bone marrow. He said he looked at ten slides and saw only one clump of neuroblastoma cells. That's one too many clumps for me! My big worry is that, although his disease seems to respond very well to active treatment, it will thrive again in full force once the treatment is stopped.

Between work and everyone's activities this week, we are running a very tight schedule. We are praying for a manageable week. Thank you to everyone in advance for your help at home and at the hospital this coming week.

Saturday, 9/25 ~ Recovering from a toxic round

Jonathan tolerated the chemo this week fairly well. He hasn't held down any food the last three to four days but hasn't had much of an appetite either. One of the side effects of one of the anti-nausea drugs he received is drowsiness, so he also slept 2-3 hours each day. Jonathan was released yesterday afternoon after receiving a red blood cell transfusion. We went straight from the hospital to the Homecoming Parade at my school because Jonathan sooo wanted to ride in the parade with his sisters. I drove down I-94 holding a bucket while Jonathan threw up beside me. But he kept telling me to drive faster because he didn't want to be late to the parade!

He seems glad to be home but still isn't keeping any food down. We had the whole family over for dinner last night, as we expect to be back in the hospital soon. Aunt Lynn and Uncle Sal brought Jonathan a bright red scooter so he could be just like Po, his favorite Teletubbie! His next blood draw is Monday.

I had a nice, long talk with Dr. Lorenzana while Jonathan and I were in the hospital on Friday. Dr. Lorenzana and Dr. Sawaf are partners, although it always seems like we run into Dr. Sawaf more often than Dr. Lorenzana. Dr. Lorenzana seemed to have time for a nice, long, casual conversation, and I appreciated his insight into our situation. More than anything, he really seemed to understand the difficulties we were facing and reminded us that there are no right or wrong answers – only choices.

Dr. Cheung from Sloan-Kettering has also suggested that we do seven days of "whole-head" radiation before the next round of chemo. Tom and I are really concerned about the side effects of "whole-head" radiation as the radiation would penetrate the brain. We plan to meet with Dr. Chuba, the radiologist, on Tuesday to discuss the actual procedure and possible side effects. I am spending much of my time reviewing current clinical trials, as we have one more round of chemo to go before we prepare to go to New York for the antibody treatment.

(I just got a call from Dr. Chuba. He had to cancel our radiology appointment. We will reschedule when he gets back in town.)

October 1999

Friday, 10/1 ~ I hate fish ...
Well, we've been home for a week now and things are approaching normal. Tom and I wanted to do something special for the kids so we took them to the pet store to pick out their very own pet—FISH!!! Goldie, Speckles, and Kitty. (Buzz named his Kitty because he really wanted a kitten!) They were so excited! Guess how many fish were floating by morning?? Mom told the kids that the fish were still sleeping and Dad did his thing. I'm not quite sure what we are going to say later today.

Sunday, 10/3 ~ Still home!
We've been home for over a week now! Can you believe it!! Jonathan always seems to defy the odds. His appetite is getting better, but he says his "body hurts." We have a blood draw scheduled for tomorrow afternoon. Tom and I both think he needs some blood products. We have truly enjoyed being "normal" for a week!!

We also found a church that we really like—Shepherd's Gate Lutheran Church in Shelby Township. The services are contemporary in style, the congregation is rather non-denominational, the music is uplifting, and we have really connected with the Pastor. (Coincidentally, Pastor Jon is also a physics major!) We have been attending most Sundays since early August. We are planning to have Jonathan and Elizabeth baptized on October 24th during the 11:30 am church service. Please join us!

Monday, 10/4 ~ Fever and low platelets

Well, right after posting the above, we headed to the hospital because of a fever – how ironic! It also looks like we spent too much time at home. Jonathan's platelet count was 4000 (again, normal is about 150,000-450,000). We finally saw those purple dots everyone looks for. After a red blood cell and platelet transfusion, however, he was back to normal. Jonathan also had a routine chest x-ray this afternoon. We call this "getting your picture taken." For some reason, the technician needed to redo his chest x-ray. We told Jonathan they had to redo the picture because he didn't smile big enough in the first one. So Jonathan climbed back up on the chair and smiled from ear to ear!! That's Jonathan, our happy child!

Tuesday, 10/5 ~ Radiation meeting

We met with Dr. Chuba and the radiology team this afternoon. Good news. The radiologists feel that the tumor sites on Jonathan's head can be treated with local radiation rather than whole-head radiation. We are sooo relieved. Jonathan will begin radiation tomorrow – twice a day for seven consecutive days. He will then be ready for his last round of chemo. After that, it is on to New York!

We have been spending much of this week confirming our choice of treatment options and trying to determine a timeline for the future. We are again gathering opinions from some of the top neuroblastoma doctors/researchers. I missed Parent-Teacher Conferences this afternoon due to the re-scheduling of the radiation meeting. I now have a number of parents to call ...

Wednesday, 10/6 ~ Pediatric décor!

Jonathan got to paint his hospital door today. (He wanted to do so for a long time.) He painted red and black blobs to go with his GO WINGS logo. It makes the room feel much more personal! The paints are still on the windowsill waiting for his next creative moment.

Saturday, 10/9 ~ Fully recovered

Jonathan's counts have fully recovered, and he seems to be feeling great. We surprised the girls last night with tickets to see "Joseph and the Amazing Technicolor Dreamcoat" at the Masonic Temple. Tom and I have both missed spending time with them. It was a GREAT show! Jonathan stayed home and enjoyed being pampered by Grandma and Grandpa D.

Thursday, 10/14 ~ Radiation therapy

After chemo, radiation is proving to be a breeze. Jonathan is remarkable! He climbs up on the table, the team marks the spot, tapes his head, covers his eyes, and he doesn't move his head an inch! He teases the radiologists, however, by wiggling his fingers that stick out from under the edge of his blanket. Radiation lasts only 20 seconds, and we were given a special parking pass, so we're in and out of the hospital within minutes. Just enough time to earn a sucker!

By the way, I have to state publicly that the St. John Hospital radiation team is absolutely wonderful!!! They have gone out of their way to make Jonathan smile and to help him relax. They know that he loves the Red Wings, so they hung Red Wings posters all around the room and on the ceiling. And each day, they give him a small gift upon leaving. Thanks to these ladies, Jonathan now has Red Wings pajamas, a "Wing Nut" hat, a Red Wings beanie baby, a Red Wings pillow, Red Wings autographed photos, and lots and lots of fruit roll-ups!! Jonathan actually enjoys "getting his picture taken!"

Thursday, 10/21 ~ Last round of chemo ...

We finished radiation on Sunday, had Monday off, and returned for chemo Tuesday morning. I took the day off; Tom went to school. Going to the hospital has become so routine, it honestly feels like a second home. We enjoy chatting with the other parents and catching up with the doctors, nurses, staff members, etc. Being that this is our last round, I have even dropped my push for outpatient chemotherapy. The chemo is progressing well, and Jonathan should be home tomorrow evening.

Again, thanks to all of you who have helped us get this far. We truly admire those who continually find time in their own lives to help others unconditionally. We have learned from you and hope that we can one day do the same for others.

Friday, 10/22 ~ A permanent reminder ...

Jonathan left his mark in the hospital playroom today by painting a ceiling tile. He also enjoyed making Halloween cookies, pumpkins, and ghosts with Sabrina (our sitter) and Sandy (St. John's Child Life Specialist). Tom brought Jonathan home this evening. He seems to be feeling ok. We are getting ready for a busy weekend ...

Sunday, 10/24 ~ Baptism

Elizabeth and Jonathan were baptized at church this morning. We were filled with emotion when Pastor Jon asked the entire congregation to pray for Jonathan and are glad that Jonathan seems to feel so comfortable around him. We had the family over for dinner after the service, and Jonathan especially enjoyed spending the day with all of his cousins. Right now, Jonathan is doing great! However, we are watching his counts …

Wednesday, 10/27 ~ Another fever …

Tom and Jonathan returned to the hospital this evening. Jonathan has low counts and a fever. Rather routine. I just hope we're home for Halloween.

Friday, 10/29 ~ Halloween at the hospital

Jonathan led the Halloween parade at this hospital this afternoon. He dressed up as Po, his favorite Teletubbie. The group went Trick-or-Treating through the halls of the hospital and received lots and lots of candy and small gifts. Jonathan, however, was not really himself. I don't think he liked the excess attention and commotion.

Saturday, 10/30 ~ Back home

Jonathan was released this morning on IV antibiotics. Actually, we threatened to break out if we weren't officially released for Halloween. The "safety" of the hospital is not worth missing this once-a-year childhood experience!

Sunday, 10/31 ~ Happy Halloween and Happy Birthday, Uncle Mike!!!

Jonathan has been very cranky the last couple of days, crying off and on, and complaining that his mouth hurts. I think he may have mouth sores from the chemo. He got them with his transplant but hasn't had them since. I hope he feels better soon. I really want him to have a great Halloween!

By the way, we had a lot of help this year putting together Halloween costumes. Thank you Aunt Laurie and Uncle Chris for Jonathan's Po costume. Thank you again to Aunt Lynn and Uncle Sal for the red Po "scootie," and many, many thanks to Halloween Fairies, Diane Maurer and Patti Ritter (co-workers), for the great Dorothy and hippie costumes for the girls!!

November 1999

Wednesday, 11/3 ~ It's always something ...
Tom took Jonathan back to the hospital this afternoon for a platelet transfusion. They should be home sometime this evening.

Saturday, 11/6 ~ Another transfusion
Jonathan had a blood draw yesterday afternoon. The doctor called this morning and said that he needs a red blood cell transfusion today. We are going to take him down later this evening and let the cells run overnight. Not going to waste a precious "day" in the hospital!

Sunday, 11/7 ~ Done with local treatment
Well, Jonathan is back home, and we are technically done with our local treatment. The good news is that the chemo and all the subsequent unplanned hospital stays are over. We are looking forward to being able to schedule treatment times and live a normal life in between. We are currently in discussions with our health insurance company as we look to begin the antibody treatments in New York soon.

Tom and I have both admitted that we are scared about the future. Truthfully, I'm on the verge of falling apart. We have come to accept the present, but so much of the future is unknown territory. Just the thought of a new hospital, new doctors, new living arrangements, etc., makes me anxious and stressed. I don't have the time or energy right now to re-establish the relationships that we have here. Also, I'm nervous about the new protocol. We know that his disease responds to chemo. What if it doesn't respond to the anti-bodies?? I want someone to tell me that we are doing the right thing and that everything will be ok. I just want to be together as a family—always and forever.

Tuesday, 11/9 ~ Baseline tests

Jonathan has a number of tests scheduled this week—a bone scan, x-rays, an EKG, CAT scan, MIBG scan, urine test, blood work-up, etc. These tests are to serve as baseline data for when he enrolls in the new study. The results of these tests will also allow us to reassess his current condition. We had some of the tests done today; the others will be completed over the next few days. The New York doctors also want to do a bone marrow aspiration, but they want this test to be done at their facility. We have this test scheduled for next Thursday, 11/18.

Because we only have this one test scheduled while in New York, we decided that this would be a good time to bring the girls to New York to let them see the city, the hospital, the Ronald McDonald house, etc. They are very excited about going and Jonathan can't wait to show them the hospital and Ronald McDonald House playrooms. We are leaving next Wednesday evening and plan to return Friday afternoon. Jonathan will then begin his treatment at MSKCC on Monday, November 29th.

Monday, 11/15 ~ One more day of tests ...

Jonathan has an ultrasound scheduled for tomorrow morning. This is the last of his scheduled tests. I called the hospital last Friday and requested a copy of all of his medical records and reports. I am picking up the packet tomorrow. I cannot wait to read all the documents! We're also preparing for this week's trip. Jonathan is counting down the days. "Just two more days till we go to New York ..."

Sunday, 11/21 ~ Summary of trip

We left for New York City last Wednesday after school. If my sister, Laurie, didn't stop by after school to see if we needed help, I don't think we would have made the plane. We flew from Detroit into Newark. We then took a cab to Manhattan and arrived at the Ronald McDonald House about 11:00 pm. We were all sleeping by 11:30 pm. We woke up early the next morning and walked the five blocks to the hospital.

The hospital visit went fairly smoothly. The hospital has a wonderful playroom staffed by a number of full-time employees and volunteer workers. The girls spent the whole time in the playroom working on crafts and playing games with the volunteers. Jonathan did the same in between blood tests, vital signs, and the bone marrow aspiration. He didn't like the doctors and nurses "interrupting" his play to do their work! Because the kids were occupied, Tom and I were able to talk freely with the doctors/researchers and the other neuroblastoma parents present. We did not learn anything new but spent over three hours with the doctors discussing Jonathan's prognosis and the antibody treatment. (I'm sure Dr. Sawaf is laughing that I'm now bothering someone else!)

The neuroblastoma research team consists of three doctors
– Dr. Cheung, Dr. Kushner, and Dr. Kramer. These doctors "live, eat, and breathe" neuroblastoma. We feel that
their guidance and expertise affords Jonathan the greatest
chance of beating this disease. Dr. Kushner is starting a
new phase II clinical trial called "Monoclonal antibody
3F8 plus oral etoposide for treatment of neuroblastoma
(MSKCC-99-33)." Many of the new neuroblastoma treatment protocols, such as the antibody treatment, attempt
to use the body's own immune system to fight recurring
disease. Past research has shown that both the monoclonal antibodies and the chemotherapy agent, etoposide
(also known as VP-16), have been somewhat successful
in treating neuroblastoma. They report that antibodies,
given after high-dose chemotherapy, have produced long-
term remissions (perhaps cures) in about 40% of first
time patients. The actual percentages for relapsed patients
such as Jonathan, however, are difficult to access and
compare due to the varying initial treatment protocols
and the increasing chemo dosages offered to first time
patients. Regardless, whatever the numbers, we were
assured that there are stage IV, relapsed patients out there
who received antibodies who are now considered long-
term survivors. Low-dose VP-16, on the other hand, has
kept a number of neuroblastoma cancers "in check" for
a period of time but has never been shown to produce a
cure on its own. Some patients choose to go on VP-16
while they "wait" for a better treatment protocol to be
developed. Dr. Kushner's new study combines these two
modalities – the monoclonal antibodies and the low-dose
VP-16. His hope is that the VP-16 will hold the cancer
at bay while the monoclonal antibodies attempt to stim-
ulate the body's immune system to produce antibodies

against the neuroblastoma cells.

Under the protocol guidelines, Jonathan will receive 10 days of antibodies the first month, and then 21 days of oral VP-16 the next month. This pattern will continue until his immune system begins making antibodies to the monoclonal antibodies. Jonathan is the third child participating in the study. The study will be closed and subsequently published after treating and following a total of 50 patients. It is so frustrating that there are no quotable statistics. I like having data, not being the data!! However, as much as this is very distressing, as a science teacher, it is also very fascinating.

We returned to the Ronald McDonald House (RMH) about 3:30 pm and checked out the playroom. The kids loved the video arcade and ping pong table. I spent my time checking out the computer lab for transmission possibilities. We went to a small restaurant a few blocks away for dinner and were back to the RMH by 6:30 pm. After enjoying some popcorn in the communal dining room, we were in bed by 9:00 pm. So much for seeing the nightlife in New York City! Friday morning, we packed, and took a cab back to Newark. Along the way, we caught a glimpse of 5th Avenue, Madison Square Garden, and the Empire State Building as we weaved through traffic. I hope we can do some sightseeing on a future trip. We caught a 12:10 pm flight and were back in Detroit by 2:00 pm. On the way home, we stopped by my school to pick up a stack of physics tests that need to be corrected. Even though we were only gone two days, I am physically and emotionally exhausted. We're preparing to return on the 28th.

Tuesday, 11/23 ~ Looking for flights

Ok, am I stupid, or what?? I spent three hours on the phone today trying to secure last minute flights to New York for Tom, Jonathan, and me for Sunday night of Thanksgiving weekend—one of the busiest travel days of the year. Impossible!! The best I could come up with was a 6:45 am flight Saturday morning into Newark. I'm not too pleased about this. I lose two days at home with the kids and my annual after-Thanksgiving holiday shopping weekend!! Tom has a return flight on Tuesday, and Jonathan and I will return ten days later, at the conclusion of his first round of antibody treatment, on 12/11.

Saturday, 11/27 ~ In New York ...

I was not happy with my alarm clock at 4:00 am this morning. The girls spent the night at Grandma D's. Tom, Jonathan, and I left the house by 5:00 am. The actual flight and arrival day was uneventful. (I didn't get sick this time!) We arrived at the RMH by 9:30 am, unpacked, and spent the afternoon relaxing and catching up on sleep.

Sunday, 11/28 ~ Sight-seeing

Well, the one good thing about getting here two days early is that we had time to do some sightseeing! Today, we visited the Statue of Liberty. Tom, Jonathan and I took a bus downtown to the southern tip of Manhattan and then took the ferry to the Statue. We had a great view of the New York skyline from the boat! We climbed the 334 steps to the pedestal, with Tom carrying Jonathan most of the way, but then quickly descended because it was getting dark. We ended up on the last boat back and didn't have time to visit Ellis Island. Tom and I would like to return when we have more time. Because we headed back so late, we were also able to enjoy the night skyline on the return trip. I think our first weekend in New York City was a success. We learned how to move around, buy groceries (you leave your cart at the "end" of the isle!), and hail a cab. I'm not sure if I could live here though. New York City is much louder, faster, and more tightly-cramped than the suburbs. I'm used to sprawling lawns, driveways, and green grass.

Monday, 11/29 ~ Day 1: An awful day

Today was the big day – our first day of the antibody treatment. We got to the hospital about 9:00 am. A nurse started pre-meds about 11:00 am – Tylenol and morphine for pain and Benedryl for allergic reactions. At this point, the meds were preventative. The Benedryl must have made Jonathan tired, as he fell asleep watching TV about 15 minutes later. After a half hour of pre-meds and hydration, the antibody infusion was started at a rate of 20 ml/hr. Jonathan slept through this. After 30 minutes, the rate was then increased to 40 ml/hr. Seconds after increasing the infusion rate, Jonathan woke up screaming in pain. He kept screaming, "Stop! Stop! I want to go home!" I just broke down and sobbed. Thankfully, Tom was there and held it together. The nurses gave him a few more doses of morphine, more Benedryl, and some Ativan to help manage the pain and calm him down. But he kicked, screamed, cried, and rolled around in pain for about half an hour before the medication seemed to ease the pain. After this half an hour, the infusion rate was then increased to 80 ml/hr, and he was given another dose of morphine, this time as a preventative measure. We were warned by the other parents that most of the children experience the greatest pain at this higher infusion rate. Surprisingly, he slept through the rest of the infusion. After the infusion ended (about one-and-a-half hours from start to finish), he slept for another hour. He woke up groggy and didn't want to go anywhere. We carefully moved him to the stroller and wheeled him back to the Ronald McDonald House five blocks away. He fell right back to sleep after starting one of his favorite videos, "How the Grinch Stole Christmas." The doctors also said that the pain meds can cause irritability. Jonathan doesn't need any help with that! He slept on and off until 6:30 pm. He woke up every now and then and complained that his feet hurt. I don't know if that was due to the meds or the antibodies. He really didn't eat all day but drank some Coke before bed.

The nurse said that this extremely, awful day was an average day ~ that some days will be better, but others may be worse. On the other hand, there were six kids here today getting antibodies. Jonathan was the only one who cried out in pain. The boy next to us played the entire time, and the others oscillated between sleeping and watching TV. The other parents tried to console us by reminding us that things will get better as the doctors figure out which pain meds are most effective for Jonathan and learn when they should be administered. We are going to try a different drug combination tomorrow and give Jonathan some Ativan up front. I hope it goes better because I cannot endure another repeat of today. I was so upset, uptight, and emotional that my stomach hurt. I also cried as I flipped the pages of a Good Housekeeping magazine. You know, all those heart-warming stories …

Tuesday, 11/30 ~ Day 2: A little bit better … maybe
Jonathan did not sleep well last night. He kept waking up and crying that his body, and especially his feet, hurt. He would fall asleep if I rubbed his body and massaged his

feet. We tried giving him a warm bath in the middle of the night but that didn't help. He finally fell asleep about 3:00 am and slept until we woke him this morning. He woke up in a great mood – his normal self – and was excited to head back to the hospital playroom. He didn't seem to remember anything about yesterday afternoon. (I forgot to mention that he got "forget" medication yesterday as well!)

We got to the hospital early this morning and let Jonathan play in the playroom while we talked to the doctors about yesterday's infusion and the after effects. They explained that the pain is very real and that they are working to develop an antibody regimen that eliminates or at least minimizes some of the pain. The pain is caused by the antibodies attaching themselves to certain proteins on the cell membrane. Because neuroblastoma cells are immature nerve cells, targeting neuroblastoma cells ultimately stimulates the nerve cells. The doctors said that many patients have complained that their feet hurt, but they didn't know what made the feet so sensitive. I asked the doctors for a prescription for a pain medication that we could give Jonathan after hours in case his body hurt again like last night. We picked up the pain med at the hospital pharmacy at the end of the day.

Jonathan's reaction to today's infusion was similar to yesterday's. It helped, however, knowing what to expect. Jonathan again began experiencing severe pain during the 40 ml/hr rate. The nurses gave him morphine every 10-15 minutes this time, but he still screamed and cried for forty-five minutes. We finally got the pain under control, and he fell asleep for the rest of the infusion. While Jonathan was sleeping, Tom and I talked. We both agreed that if the pain could not be better managed, we would consider removing Jonathan from the study. We're going to talk to the doctors about this tomorrow morning.

Tom left the hospital mid-afternoon today to catch a cab back to Newark. He had a 4:30 pm flight that ended up being delayed until 6:00 pm. He got home about 9:00 pm. Now it's just me and Jonathan. Mom always has the best ideas though – the candy store, the ice cream shop, FAO Schwartz, etc. They're all waiting for us!

December 1999

Wednesday, 12/1 ~ Day 3: Just me and Buzz
This is starting to become routine. We get up about 7:30 am, get ready to go, pack the stroller, buy two Cokes from the twenty-five cent pop machine at the RMH, start walking the five blocks to the hospital, stop at a street vendor for coffee and bagels, chase the pigeons along the way, and arrive at the hospital by 9:00 – 9:30 am. I check in while Jonathan runs straight to the playroom. While Jonathan plays and/or participates in the daily activity, I chat with the other moms. Patient names are called over the PA system when it is that person's turn to be seen in the clinic. Every time an announcement is made, Jonathan stops and listens closely. Most times, he responds, "That not my neeme!" and immediately goes back to playing. When they do call his name, he jumps up and says, "That my neeme!! Let go, Momma!!" So he doesn't seem to be too bothered by the treatment regime.

We are usually called to the bed area of the clinic about 10:00 – 10:30 am. Jonathan willingly takes his pre-meds and pops in a video. We watch "Frosty the Snowman," "How the Grinch Stole Christmas" (and he yells at the Grinch to "take the tree back" every time!), "Kiki's Delivery Service," and "The Brave Little Toaster Goes to Mars" over and over. I still haven't figured out why a toaster goes to Mars ...

Today's antibody treatment seemed to go slightly better than yesterday's. (Things are either getting better or perhaps I just know better what to expect.) Jonathan cried for about 45 minutes during the end of the infusion but fell asleep by 1:00 pm. He then slept off/on until around 7:00 pm. I relaxed and read magazines – something I rarely have time to do these days.

We used a different pain med today. Instead of morphine, Jonathan received Dilaudid. This seemed to better control his pain. Jonathan received a dose of Dilaudid each time the rate was increased even if he wasn't showing any outward signs of pain. I think this helped keep the pain under control for a longer period of time. He didn't experience pain today until the end of the 80 ml/hr infusion rate. Two more doses of Dilaudid and he slept the rest of the afternoon. He hasn't experienced any more foot pain, but tonight Jonathan complained about a headache for most of the evening. The doctor on call said that the headache was most likely due to the Dilaudid. We spent the evening in our room at the RMH with Jonathan playing cars and me catching up on my email.

Thursday, 12/2 ~ Day 4: A new room

They moved us to a new room today. The usual bed area of the clinic has a circle of beds about two feet apart from one another – not a lot of space or privacy. Because

Jonathan has been having such a difficult time (translation, crying so much), they moved us to a little side room. This room was once a small office, but it now houses two beds. We were there by ourselves. I like the quietness and privacy. There was nothing special about treatment today. We seemed to have found a routine that works for Jonathan. He still seems to experience some pain near the end of the transfusion but, after another dose of pain med, he soon falls asleep for the rest of the afternoon.

Lunch is served every day in the clinic to anyone who is there. As always, Jonathan gets excited about the food but then eats nothing. He instead asks for a Happy Meal as we pass McDonalds on the walk home from the hospital. He usually ends up eating the cold Happy Meal about 9:00 pm back at the RMH when he is feeling better. He actually likes cold (and even frozen!) chicken nuggets.

More good news ... my sister, Laurie, arrived this evening. After traveling alone and then taking a cab to an address scribbled on a piece of paper, she said she was relieved to see a familiar face when she got off the elevator on the ninth floor of the RMH. We went out for a late dinner (Jonathan complained of a headache most of the time), toured the Ronald McDonald House, and played in the playroom. I'm looking forward to her company at the hospital tomorrow.

Friday, 12/3 ~ Day 5: A great day!
I can't believe it! Jonathan didn't experience any pain today! He still received medication as the infusion rate was increased, but the meds seemed to control and/or prevent the pain. He slept peacefully through the afternoon and, all

in all, received less medication than in previous days. Laurie and I spent the day talking and just relaxing. Interestingly, some of the other children receiving antibodies also did not experience any pain today. I don't know what to think. I'm thrilled that Jonathan had a great day, but it makes me wonder if something was wrong with the antibodies today.

Because Jonathan received less medication today, he was back to his normal self by dinner time. Laurie and I decided we should hit the town! We took a cab to Rockefeller Center – well, we tried to – but there where so many people in the area that we instead jumped out of the cab and walked the last few blocks, pushing Jonathan in the stroller. You would never guess it was December in New York City. The weather was unseasonably warm and absolutely beautiful! We admired the Christmas tree, ran into Santa (Jonathan told Santa the only thing he wants for Christmas is a whistle), looked for "Good Morning America," then walked up 5th Avenue. New York City is awesome! We decided we would walk until we were tired and then take a cab home from wherever we were. Before we knew it, we were blocks from the Ronald McDonald House. We ended up walking for hours tonight! After a week in the hospital, it felt great to walk, be outdoors, and feel the spirit of holiday season.

Sunday, 12/5 ~ NYC: Been there; done that!
Laurie, Jonathan, and I had a wonderful weekend! Buzz was feeling great and the weather was absolutely beautiful all weekend! We spent most of the time out and about. Yesterday, we took a bus down toward the Statue of Liberty. Jonathan wanted fine cuisine for brunch – McDonald's chicken nuggets and french fries glopped in ketchup. We then visited the South SeaPort Mall – a quaint shopping mall

on the East River. Laurie bought a Hot Watch. (That's a joke. I couldn't get her to buy a watch from the shady men down by the ferry. She said their briefcases looked suspicious.) We had a great lunch and enjoyed adult drinks at Uno's Pizzeria. After shopping, we took the ferry to the Statue of Liberty (again!) and then went on to Ellis Island. By the time we finished looking around the island, it was dark. We ended up again on the last boat back from the island. Jonathan was worried that the boat wasn't going to come back to get us (and the other hundred people waiting in line.) We caught the M-15 Limited (the best bus!) and Jonathan fell asleep on Laurie's lap within minutes. We went back to the RMH, rested for a bit, and then went downstairs to the playroom where Jonathan played arcade games and made gingerbread houses before going to bed. Laurie and I commented on how cool it was to look out the windows of the RMH and see the bright city lights of Manhattan.

We woke up Sunday morning with renewed energy and motivation. We had another fun-filled day of great plans. We went out for breakfast and then headed to the World Trade Center. (I bought a fake leather coat for Elizabeth yesterday at the Gap at the South SeaPort Mall, but they didn't have one in Melissa's size. We tracked one down for Melissa at the Gap in the World Trade Center.) Of course the World Trade Center is back near the southern tip of Manhattan but on the West Side—not a direct hike from where we were in Midtown on the East Side. Laurie studied the bus routes and got us there with minimal transfers. We walked around the World Trade Center, took a few pictures to prove we were there, found the Gap, purchased the jacket, and then headed back to the shopping district. We visited the Empire State Building, Macy's department store, and shopped along 5th Avenue. Before we knew it, it was again dark. We especially liked The Disney Store, Warner Brothers, and FAO Schwarz. (The 2nd floor Barbie section of FAO Schwarz even emanates a pink hue on the sidewalk below.) And the window displays along 5th Avenue – specially decked out for Christmas – were truly spectacular! We ended our day with a horse and buggy ride through Central Park in the dark and then watched the ice skaters skating on the rink below. Jonathan was the only one left with any energy.

Monday, 12/6 ~ Day 6: Back to the hospital

Laurie headed back home this morning. She caught a cab on our way to the hospital. (Of course it was pouring down rain and cabs were few and far between.) As she pulled away, I stood there on the corner crying in the rain. I don't like being here by myself. I quickly got myself together and continued walking to the hospital. Jonathan fell right back into his normal routine – check in, Monday morning poke and vitals, then off to the playroom! The antibody treatment was much like last week. Jonathan experienced pain during the end of the 80 ml/hr infusion rate, but we were able to keep it under control. I'm glad that my brother, Michael, is due to arrive later this evening.

Tuesday, 12/7 ~ Day 7: Getting routine

Jonathan loves having Uncle Mike with him at the hospital. They made snowflakes at the craft table, played a few games of pool, and checked out the board games, cars, toys, books, and videos. Again, treatment went fairly smoothly. Jonathan received pain meds throughout the infusion, but again only seemed uncomfortable near the end. I really enjoyed having a chance to catch up with Michael. Because he lives in

Washington, D.C., we rarely get a chance to spend this kind of time together. It is also very helpful to have a second person around to help locate doctors, nurses, lunch, etc. Michael and I had a nice, long talk with Dr. Cheung today. I'm glad Michael got to meet him. We spent the evening hours in the RMH playroom.

Wednesday, 12/8 ~ Day 8: Hospital Christmas Party
Today was the hospital Christmas Party. As a result, treatment for all children was delayed so that everyone could attend the morning festivities. The playroom hosted a professional juggler who juggled anything and everything (and concluded with very long, sharp knives), a Christmas sing-a-long, and holiday snacks. Jonathan wasn't entertained by the juggler or the sing-a-long. He just wanted to play pool with Uncle Mike. It is soooo helpful that he looks forward to going to the hospital each day! (Note to hospital administrators: Never underestimate the value of a wonderful playroom!)

Treatment went well again today. He received pain meds throughout the infusion, but this time, was alert and coherent throughout the treatment. I thought we were going to make it through pain-free, but today he experienced pain after the infusion finished. He soon fell asleep and slept the rest of the afternoon. I'm getting tired of reading magazines …

Thursday, 12/9 ~ Day 9: Almost done!
Michael left this morning. He caught a cab on our morning walk to the hospital. Again, I cried at the corner. (At least it wasn't raining this time.) I stopped to visit the "bagel man." I owed him a dime from yesterday. Jonathan gives

him a hard time each morning as he picks out his donut. "I want the pink one. No, the frosted one. No, the one with sprinkles," all while the New York City rush hour pedestrians line up behind him. Jonathan played in the playroom then picked out the same four videos. Nurse Karen always stops in and watches "Frosty" with Jonathan. She said it is her favorite video too. (By the way, Jonathan loves Nurse Karen!) Treatment went fairly well. Again, Jonathan didn't experience any pain until after the infusion ended. Then he complained that his body hurt for about a half hour and then fell asleep. I spent my time asking questions and securing discharge instructions so we can leave tomorrow as soon as possible.

When we got back to the RMH, I was so excited. I cannot wait to go home!! I miss Tom. I miss the girls. I miss our family. I miss my house, my job, Michigan, grass, trees, open space, peace and quiet, birds chirping, and everything New York is not!

So Jonathan and I started packing. I wanted to have everything stacked and ready to go so that when we leave the hospital tomorrow, we can immediately catch a cab to the airport. Jonathan and I packed and packed. With all of our shopping, we have more to take home than we came with, and I will be all by myself at the airport. By 7:00 pm I had all the boxes taped closed and ready to go. I just wanted to lie in bed and watch TV. But no, Jonathan said he was "bored." He started pulling the tape off the box of his toys. "No, Jonathan!!!!," I said. "We cannot unpack all the toys!!!" So now what? There wasn't much to do. It was raining outside, the RMH playroom was closed, and I didn't want him to start unpacking boxes. So I suggested we take a walk down to the dining room. I had read in the lobby that a local Italian restaurant was catering tonight's dinner and there was supposed to be a Christmas Party afterwards. Wow! I can't believe tonight's events. The dinner was excellent—not just Italian food, but fine Italian cuisine. Then as we were finishing dinner, guess who showed up? Frosty the Snowman!!!! When Frosty walked in Jonathan stopped in his tracks, and his eyes lit up. After two weeks of watching Frosty on video, he couldn't believe that he was now actually here in the flesh (well, perhaps costume). Jonathan ran across the room and threw his arms around Frosty. As Frosty moved, Jonathan clung to his waist. (He was very round!) I had to pry him off after a few minutes. Every time I turned around, however, Jonathan was back hanging on Frosty—literally! As Frosty made his way to the door, with Jonathan not far behind, Santa Claus made his grand entrance. Jonathan just stood there in awe, not knowing who was grander. Santa then asked all the families to go down a floor to the Living Room area for the Annual Ronald McDonald House Christmas Party. The party was co-sponsored by Pepsi-Cola and Macy's department store. You would not believe the gifts that were handed out. Santa called each child up, one by one, talked with them, and then showered them with gifts. Jonathan received a five foot stocking stuffed with toys (balls, games, cars, craft kits, puzzles, squirt guns, etc.) and a large Macy's shopping bag filled with more toys and stuffed animals. Each parent was also given a large box of Christmas ornaments from Macy's, a beautiful Radio City Music Hall snow globe, and a large set of Nutcracker figurines. Later that night, Macy's bags were delivered to each child's room with gifts for each of his or her siblings. So I inherited two more large bags of toys, one for Melissa and one for Elizabeth. The evening concluded with a raffle in which we won a stereo component in a big, big box. I stood there looking at the huge pile of goods sitting in front of us and thought just one thing: "How am I going to get all of this stuff home?" And I also have two large suitcases, a stroller, two large boxes of toys, a portable TV/VCR combo unit, and Jonathan who likes to be carried. My anxiety level is increasing.

Friday, 12/10 ~ Day 10: Going home!!
I got up early today, cleaned the room, and washed the linens. (There is no housekeeping service at the RMH!) I told the nurses yesterday that I would like to start as early as possible today so that Jonathan would have maximum time to recover before our evening flight. We got to the hospital at 9:30 am, and they had already called Jonathan's name. Jonathan immediately started his pre-meds and spent just a few minutes in the playroom. He doesn't seem particularly excited about going home. Again, treatment went fairly well—just some minor pain during the last half hour of the infusion. We got back to the RMH by 4:00 pm. I did some last minute packing, and we grabbed a quick dinner. By 5:30 pm, we were ready to go. It took me three trips to get everything down to the lobby. Of course, as luck would have it, it was now pouring down rain. The chipper (that's sarcastic!) desk clerk wished me luck finding a cab during rush hour in the rain on a Friday night in New York with lots and lots of stuff. Guess I lucked out. Jonathan and I walked down a block and quickly hailed a cab. I had the cab driver circle around and stop in front of the RMH to pick up our stuff. It filled the whole cab—front seat, back seat, laps, and trunk!!! I sat in the back holding Jonathan (because he wanted to see out the window) with three Macy's shopping bags full of toys blocking our view! The cab driver

then helped me get everything to the baggage check at the airline ticket counter. I checked the suitcases, boxes, stroller, TV, etc. and just kept the shopping bags. Jonathan and I picked up something to eat and relaxed at the gate. Our flight left on time from Newark at 8:55 pm. Luckily, the plane was only half-full, and surprisingly, we were upgraded to first class. I leaned my head against the window and was enjoying the low lights, peaceful night, and quiet flight. Of course that didn't last. Halfway through the flight, Jonathan started singing Jingle Bells in a very, very loud voice. As I tried to quiet him down, those around us started singing along. Soon, everyone on the plane was singing along! After a few more sing-along Christmas songs, Jonathan was looking for something else to do. I was so tired, and Jonathan seemed to have more and more energy. Next thing I know, he accidentally ripped the shopping bags and three soccer balls went rolling down the aisle of the plane. I am sure that our unsuspecting antics either humored or annoyed those who were lucky enough to share our flight! By the time we landed, I had retrieved the balls but now had a pile of ripped bags and a lot of loose toys. So Jonathan got off the plane in Detroit carrying one soccer ball while Mom carried two ~ and everything else. Jonathan ran through the jetway and immediately saw Tom in the distance. He ran as fast as he could yelling, "Daddy, Daddy! Let play soccer!!" So at 11:30 pm, Tom and Jonathan were kicking the soccer ball back and forth in the airport terminal. Jonathan missed his Daddy so much. Ohhh, it feels soooo good to be home!!

Sunday, 12/12 ~ Getting re-acclimated

Although it feels great to be home, I'm having a hard time getting re-acclimated. I feel like I am living two completely different lives. Although we were only in New York for two weeks, we developed a totally different kind of routine. In New York, as soon as you walk out the door, you are in the heart of the city – block after block of tall buildings, restaurants, and store fronts. I loved the energy, the excitement, the people, and the noise. It is a fast-moving city and I felt drawn into its pace. It is such a contrast to our quiet, suburban neighborhood with large homes, sprawling yards, long driveways, and meandering roads. I actually think I could love both lifestyles, but it feels odd to oscillate between the two. Jonathan, on the other hand, adjusted within minutes and doesn't seem to mind where he plays!

Sunday, 12/19 ~ Back to school

This has been a very difficult week. I went back to school on Monday, after being gone for two weeks, and was disappointed to hear that all had not gone smoothly while I was gone. (I pre-planned all of my lessons, videotaped myself teaching some of them, had a responsible student assistant in each class, communicated via email with students and sub each evening, etc.) But I came back to issues and complaints. So-and-so was rude to the sub. Some students complained that they didn't understand the material. Some didn't like that I was gone for two whole weeks. Others were upset about their test scores, etc. One father even complained to the principal. While their comments are understandable, I also think some of them are just easy excuses. I truly appreciate that our Personnel Director is so understanding and willing to work with me. Things seemed to calm down by the end of the week after I had a chance to review some of the more difficult material and update the students as to Jonathan's progress.

Saturday, 12/25 ~ Mixed holiday feelings

It is late Christmas Eve and I seem to be lacking in holiday spirit. We celebrated Christmas with my side of the family at Laurie and Chris's earlier this evening. While we had a wonderful evening, I have so many mixed feelings. I feel like I have missed much of the holiday season here at home. While I was gone, Tom and the girls put up the tree, decorated the house, did a lot of the Christmas shopping, and made most of the holiday plans. These are the things that I normally do and enjoy. Somehow not being part of the preparation is making me feel like I missed Christmas this year. In the back of my mind, I also cannot help but think that this might be Jonathan's last Christmas. It's hard to enjoy the holiday when such a cloud of doubt hangs from above.

Sunday, 12/26 ~ Santa comes through!

As much as we wanted to shower Jonathan with gifts this year, his wish list was very short. All he wanted was a whistle. (He is fascinated by sports referees at the moment!) Luckily, Santa came through!! Everything else he received also had something to do with sports. He's definitely Daddy's little boy!! We celebrated Christmas with the Dilibertis today and are now enjoying just being home as a family.

Monday, 12/27 ~ Start oral chemo

Jonathan began taking his oral chemotherapy today. He has to squirt the chemo from a syringe and then drink the liquid three times a day. From the look on his face, I'm guessing it tastes really bad. Jonathan also had a blood draw at our local clinic this afternoon. His blood sample will be shipped to New York to be tested for a positive response to the antibodies. We won't know the results for a few days.

Friday, 12/31 ~ New Year's Eve

As 1999 comes to a close, I am reflecting on what is important in life and how far we've come. Jonathan is just a normal three-year old with some misguided cells. He embraces each new day and has no idea that he is fighting a serious disease. It has been ten months since his initial diagnosis, and our lives are forever changed. But life is what you make it. Happy New Year, everyone!

January 2000

Tuesday, 1/4 ~ Taking my med!

Jonathan continues to take the oral chemo three times a day. He has developed a routine – more like a ritual – before each dose. Pour a little pop in a cup. Squirt the med from the syringe into the pop. Put the empty syringe in the red jug. Make sure Mom is standing very nearby. Drink some "good" pop from the can, eat some chocolate, gulp the med, drink some more pop, then wash it all down with a frozen chicken nugget. I wonder how closely Jonathan's regime compares with the original treatment protocol!

Sunday, 1/16 ~ Last day of Round 1

Today was Jonathan's last day of oral chemo. He was thrilled when I told him that he didn't have to drink any more of the yucky stuff for a long time. We are scheduled to start Round Two of the antibodies on Monday, January 24th. Tom and I decided that the trip will be much easier to manage if we each spend a week with Jonathan in New York. After the first week of treatment, we will fly home on Friday and then fly back on Sunday for week two. Doing so will also allow us to spend some quality family time on Saturday, and Jonathan will just rack up some extra frequent flyer miles. Right now, the plan is for me to go the first week with my parents, and for Tom to go back the second week with his Dad.

Monday, 1/17 ~ WHAT?!?!?!?

I called MSKCC today to confirm the dates of our arrival. The receptionist paused and then said that the antibody clinical trial has been "suspended." What?!?!? What is going on?!? I am totally confused, extremely upset, and utterly frantic! I know that Jonathan has to be receiving some sort of treatment or his cancer is going to continue to spread!!!!! I couldn't get any information from anyone in New York other than that the clinical trial has been "suspended by the FDA," and that we wouldn't be receiving antibodies anytime soon. I called and left a message with our local doctors, Dr. Sawaf and Dr. Lorenzana, to see if they knew anything or if they could offer any advice.

Thursday, 1/20 ~ Still don't know ...

I spent hours on the phone and online the last few days trying to find out what is going on. No one in New York is talking, and I can't figure out "who" the FDA really is. The trial suspension is a very hot topic on my listserv at the moment. Many of the parents in this group also have children who are being treated at MSKCC. Some of the moms are talking about camping out on the FDA's doorstep in Washington D.C. until they receive an explanation. It doesn't seem right that a study, in which you are a participant (piece of data!), can be "suspended" without telling you why. I called and canceled our flights. I really don't know what to do right now ...

PART THREE

A New Normal

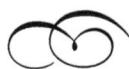

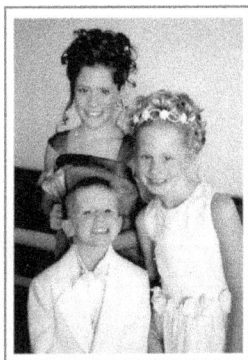

We never did learn why the antibody trial was suspended, but it quickly resumed. (Rumor was that the problem was paperwork-related.) At this point I stopped posting daily entries in the journal. Without the intense chemo and unplanned hospital stays, life at home began to feel a bit like normal—that is, if drinking chemo out of a cup for 21 days in a row can be considered "normal." We liked that treatments were now confined to a two-week period every other month, and in between, we embraced the routines of everyday life. We even enjoyed a few perks!

Make-A-Wish Trip
(2/19/00-2/25/00)

In between the second and third antibody treatments, we took our Make-A-Wish Trip. Jonathan's wish was to take a hot air balloon to meet Mickey Mouse. The Make-A-Wish folks translated that into the classic Make-A-Wish Trip to Disney World in Florida—via a plane. Luckily, we were able to schedule the trip over Winter Break; Tom and girls were off that week and I missed just three days of school. We were also thrilled that Laurie and Chris, Lynn and Sal, and their kids, were able to make arrangements to join us for the week.

The Wish trip was truly amazing. Our vacation started when a limo arrived at our home at 5:00 am to take us to the airport. The driver was quick to point out the pop, candy bars, fruit, juice, bagels, and snacks waiting for the kids in the back of the limo. They climbed in, giggled, and enjoyed a high-sucrose breakfast on the hour drive to the airport. Once in Florida, a shuttle driver met us at the airport and drove us to "Give Kids the World" – a 70-acre resort village designed to provide "memorable, magical, cost-free experiences to children with life-threatening illnesses and their families." While there, we learned that the village was designed by Walt Disney himself and has served as home to thousands of families from around the world, many on Wish trips similar to ours.

Give Kids the World looked just like Candy Land-come-to-life with its childlike curvy, paver walkways and colorful, pastel villas. The heart of the village consists of the "House of Hearts" which provides Guest Services, the "Castle of Miracles" where you can meet the Disney characters, the "Ice Cream Palace" where free ice cream is available all day long, and the "Gingerbread House" where breakfast, lunch, and dinner is served for all village residents. Village activities include horseback riding, putt-putt golf, a fishing pond, swimming at the "Park of Dreams," and nightly shows. The kiddie passenger train that meanders through the village completes the fairytale look. Day after day families are showered with gifts, surprises, and real-life Disney magic.

Upon checking in at the House of Hearts, Jonathan was given a Mickey Mouse stuffed animal. Jonathan's eyes just sparkled. From that moment on, Mickey became a prized possession—his status quickly elevating to that of the blue baby blanket. Now, everywhere we went, Jonathan carried both Mickey and vee-vee. Vee-vee was generally wadded in a ball in one arm while Mickey was carried in a head lock under the other.

For the next four days we did the Disney thing—visited Magic Kingdom, Epcot Center, Animal Kingdom, and Universal Studios. We ate breakfast most mornings at the Gingerbread House, often stopping for an ice cream along the way. (Jonathan always had the biggest grin on his face knowing he was having ice cream for breakfast!) While we were at the Disney parks, Jonathan wore a button pinned to his shirt that identified him as a "Make-A-Wish/Give Kids the World" kid. The button afforded Jonathan (and our entire group) a number of special privileges. He and the kids were always "next in line" on the rides; we were given front row seats at all of the shows, and when they were looking for audience volunteers, members of our group were always selected. Uncle Sal and Uncle Chris did a great Tarzan Yell at the Tarzan show. The kids enjoyed playing instruments and dancing in the Lion King Show, and Uncle Chris was an awesome drummer in the Doug Live Show at Universal Studios. We were a little uncomfortable with the excess attention and special treatment, but it truly made for a once-in-a-lifetime experience!

Jonathan loved everything about Disney. He loved seeing the characters, was excited about all the rides (Test Track at Epcot Center was his favorite!), and loved the singing and dancing at the shows. He especially enjoyed sharing the experience with his sisters and cousins.

I remember one afternoon, Jonathan "shared" more than expected. While at Animal Kingdom, Jonathan wanted to

start the day with a water ride—not a good idea because
Jonathan does not like his clothes to be wet or spotted! We
explained that if he went on the water ride, he would most
likely get wet and that we didn't bring a change of clothes.
But he wouldn't give up. He said he really, really, really
wanted to go on the water ride and that he "don't caa-aare"
if he got wet. Tom and I looked at each other with that "it's
his WISH trip look" and relented. Of course, he and
Elizabeth got drenched! Immediately after, while walking
to the Tarzan Show, he started complaining about being
wet. Then, as we were waiting in line for the show to start,
a woman tapped me on the shoulder and said, "Uh, excuse
me, Miss, but …" as she pointed to Jonathan. There was
Jonathan, standing next to me, completely naked with his
clothes in a pile at his feet. He explained that he couldn't
wear his clothes because "they were wet." So Tom ran off
looking for the closest booth to buy Jonathan some dry
clothes—exactly what we said we weren't going to do.
Jonathan spent the rest of the day with his button pinned
to his new, adult-sized, Tarzan t-shirt.

On our last day at Give Kids the World, we visited the
Castle of Miracles. At the end of each child's stay, a small
gold star—engraved with the child's name and age—is placed
on the ceiling of the castle. Jonathan's star was barely visible
as it was hidden among the thousands of stars already there.
We are truly humbled and especially grateful to the countless donors and anonymous volunteers who help make such
Wish trips possible.

Treatment in New York

In between life as normal, we continued to travel back
and forth to Memorial Sloan Kettering every eight weeks

or so for the antibody treatments. Jonathan had his second round of treatment in February, and completed his fifth by July. The pain experienced during the first round soon became manageable and the trips to New York actually became somewhat enjoyable. Jonathan still liked to pack his own bag – filled with toys, sleep shirts, and many stuffed friends – and would wear his Red Wings jersey as much as possible to razz all the Rangers fans in New York City. In Jonathan's eyes, the trips to New York were also enhanced by the various modes of transportation. He loved taking airplanes, buses, and subway trains, and especially loved riding in the loud "fancy yellow cars" (beat up taxis) found only in New York! Tom and I continued to take turns traveling to New York and, invariably, one of our family members would fly out to join us. By the end of the fifth round of treatment, Jonathan enjoyed visits from Aunt Laurie, Uncle Mike, Grandma and Grandpa E, Grandpa D, Aunt Laura, and Uncle Tim.

We all have very fond memories of our time in New York. When I was with Jonathan, we seemed to do a lot of shopping. We rented his favorite movies on the way to the hospital each week, stopped for chicken nuggets daily on the walk home, and went out shopping again most evenings after the days' meds wore off. We visited Jonathan's favorite candy shop, looked for small gifts for the girls, and just enjoyed being out on the town. One day, Jonathan said he needed a new "friend" as he looked up at a shelf of beanie babies in the candy shop. He chose Grover, the blue trash-can lover from Sesame Street. He now had three most important things – Mickey, vee-vee, and Grover.

When Tom was in New York, he and Jonathan enjoyed an excessive amount of sports. The Ronald McDonald House often received tickets to a variety of events which they posted daily. The desk clerk soon learned of Tom and Jonathan's love of sports and routinely offered them complimentary tickets. Tom and Jonathan watched the Rangers play with Uncle Mike, took in a New Jersey Devils and Yankees game with Grandpa D, and then saw the Mets play with Uncle Tim – not to mention the countless hours of sports on TV I'm sure they watched!

Jonathan also loved entertaining family members when they came to visit. When giving tours of the Ronald McDonald House, he always walked slowly down the basement stairs and said fearfully, "He can eat you!" as he pointed to each of the large animals painted on the stairway wall. Once in the basement, he would excitedly point out the toys, craft table, ping pong table, computer lab, and arcade games. He also loved the life-sized Tic-Tac-Toe board in the lobby – always stopping to play a game when passing through. He especially loved yelling, "Tic tac toe! Three-in-a-row!" when playing with Uncle Tim! He then led visitors on the walk to the hospital and delighted in chasing the pigeons and showing them around the hospital as well. At the hospital, Jonathan's relationship with Nurse Karen continued to flourish even though she didn't know it. Jonathan would often come home and make pictures for Nurse Karen and looked forward to seeing her upon his return. Aunt Laura, who always has good ideas, helped Jonathan pick out a bouquet of tulips for Nurse Karen from a street vendor on one of their walks to the hospital in early spring.

Even in New York, Jonathan was generally his normal, happy, chatty self. Uncle Tim recalls one long, particularly chatty taxi ride in which he and Tom made up the "Quiet Game" to see who could remain quiet the longest. It was the one game that Jonathan could not win!

At Home

The best time of all, however, was our time at home. We were finally starting to feel like a family again, and other than the 21 days of drinking the oral chemo, Jonathan was a normal 4-year-old child. He played outside, attended preschool, and participated in a sports league at a local indoor sports center. The girls continued taking piano and dance lessons, and Tom and I finally started to relax. Wow – maybe we were one of the lucky few! We continued to keep in touch with the doctors and staff at St. John Hospital and even attended their Cancer Survivor's Day picnic in mid-July.

After five rounds of antibody treatments, however, Jonathan's immune system still hadn't produced the desired response. This was not necessarily unexpected or alarming. Because the antibody treatment was still so new, and because every child responds so differently, the doctors could not predict when, or even if, Jonathan's body would eventually produce the desired anti-antibodies. The MSKCC protocol consisted of up to ten antibody treatments. So we were still patiently waiting ...

The culminating event of the summer was Dan (Tom's brother) and Nicole's wedding during Labor Day weekend. Jonathan had a special affection for Nicole and liked to call her Colie. Dan and Nicole went out of their way to include all of their nieces and nephews in their wedding party. It was a beautiful wedding!! Jonathan wore a white tuxedo and walked down the aisle with his "best bud," cousin Samantha. Melissa was a junior bridesmaid, and Elizabeth wore a white dress that matched the other "angel" cousins. Everything was just perfect. We were all together again, and everyone was having a great time – just like it used to be.

One of my most favorite memories of the night was danc-ing to "You'll be in my Heart" by Phil Collins in a large cir-cle with the whole family and all of the cousins. It is one of Jonathan's favorite songs! At the end of the night, even though Jonathan's shirt was crooked and un-tucked and we all looked a bit disheveled, we asked the photographer to take our family's picture. After a most wonderful day, the family portrait is one of our favorites!

Soon after the wedding, it was time for another set of routine scans. As always, it took days to complete all the tests and the results came in a few at a time. After almost nine months of semi-normalcy, we were anxious to receive a full report. We were also a bit nervous because Tom confided that he thought he saw a few yellow spots on the monitor during the MIBG scan …

September 22, 2000

It was late Friday afternoon, and I was still at school. I had been trying to get hold of Dr. Sawaf at St. John Hos-pital off and on throughout the day. He returned my call at 4:00 pm, and I was paged to the Main Office to take the call. I could tell that Dr. Sawaf had something to say, and that he would have preferred to speak to us in person. But it was late in the day, and I told him that we surely didn't want to wait until Monday to hear the results. I assured him that we have been through enough that I could handle any news he had to share over the phone. With a short pause and a tender voice, he then told me what I already knew. Jonathan's cancer was back … again. Upon hearing the words, however, my stomach dropped and tears imme-diately started rolling down my cheeks.

The Most Difficult Decision in the World

I don't think I slept all weekend. Every time I looked at Jonathan, tears filled my eyes. We knew in our hearts that we were losing the battle and that we were out of viable options. After a heart-felt discussion with the doctors at St. John Hospital and the researchers in New York, we made the most difficult decision of our lives – there would be no more aggressive treatment. Without aggressive treatment, the cancer would continue to spread ... until it could spread no more. With the help of hospice and palliative care, we wanted to let Jonathan just be Jonathan for as long as possible.

PART FOUR

Facing Reality

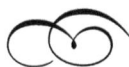

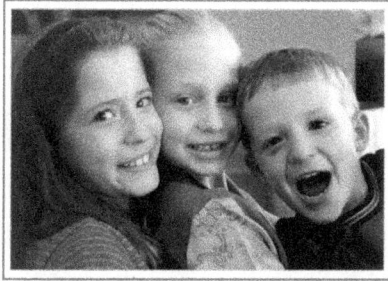

September 2000

Saturday, 9/23 ~ Telling the family

I just cannot believe this news. Although we suspected that something was going on, I cannot believe that the disease is so far advanced. Hospice called this morning, and I did not call back. Jonathan just seems so ... normal. In fact, right now, he is in the basement playing hockey! We are just so sad and so full of questions. How are we going to handle this? What, when, and how should we tell the girls? What is going to happen? What is happening inside his little body?? How many more months/weeks/days do we have?? And what about Jonathan???

Laurie and I went out this afternoon and ran a few errands. We also made arrangements to get all of the kids' pictures taken tomorrow. We want a picture with all of the cousins together. I also called and canceled our flights to New York. We cannot continue with the antibodies now that he has progressive disease. Said another way, we were kicked off the study.

We had our families over for dinner tonight and shared the news and prognosis with the adults. We all seem to have similar questions and concerns, and are worried about how the kids will react. Tom and I are going to consult with a child psychologist early this week to ask for advice on sharing this news with the kids. The cousins played together all night, and it was nice to be able to sit and talk with the rest of the family during that time.

Sunday, 9/24 ~ Special day in church

It has been quite a day. We went to church this morning, and I was very emotional. I cried through most of the service. Jonathan, on the other hand, seemed to have a special day in church. While walking out of church, Jonathan tugged on my shirt and whispered, "Momma, God talked to me today." I stopped and looked at him with a nod that said, "What?" He repeated himself and said that God talked to him while we were greeting those seated around us. Funny thing is, I do remember seeing him sitting oddly on his chair, slowly swinging his legs back and forth, looking somewhat preoccupied during this time. He didn't offer the contents of the conversation (and I didn't ask), but he seemed very content with whatever God said.

After church, we met the rest of the family at the mall for our family photo. The kids all wore blue jeans and white t-shirts. I spent the hour in between church and the photo session running around town trying to find matching white shirts in all different sizes. We got a picture of all of the cousins together; pictures of Melissa, Elizabeth, and Jonathan together; and then some of just Jonathan by himself. Jonathan wanted to wear his Red Wings jersey for his picture.

Hospice also called again today. I'm still not ready to return their call.

Monday, 9/25 ~ Just want to be Mom

Tom and I talked over the weekend and agreed it would be best if I took a leave of absence from work. Deciding which of us would continue to work or stay with Jonathan has always been a delicate balance between needs, wants, and responsibilities. Continuing to work allowed us to maintain our medical benefits and, ultimately, keep our kids' lives as normal as possible. Right now, however, I feel a strong urge to just be Mom. I want to get the girls off to school in the morning, make Jonathan breakfast, and just spend as much time with him as possible. I told a few people at school today of my intentions. I know that everyone shares in my sadness. I stayed up until 3:00 am last night doing school work.

Donna, our sitter, took Jonathan to preschool today. He is starting to love school. Hospice also called again this morning and caught me at school. I politely informed the caller that everything seemed to be progressing just fine at the moment and that I didn't feel that we needed their services at this time. She listened politely, but I sensed that she thought we should be scheduling our assessment visit. I told her I would call her back next week.

Something else happened today that still has me a bit shaken. I was sitting at my desk in the den with Jonathan coloring at my feet. Holding his crayon, he looked up at me and said, "God talks to me, you know." I looked at him, but didn't know quite how to respond. After a brief pause, trying not to sound surprised or alarmed, I said, "He does?

When does God talk to you?" Still coloring, he replied, "When I'm in my room playing cars." Then he continued, "I'm going to die, you know." "Well, everyone eventually dies, Jonathan," I added casually. "Yes. But I'm going to die pretty soon." As he continued to color, my eyes gazed deep into him, and my heart just melted. He knows he's going to die! And God talks to him!! I don't know which I'm more startled about. Something is going on.

Tuesday, 9/26 ~ Visit with child psychologist
I stayed up late again last night catching up on some school work and writing another "Jonathan Update" to our friends and neighbors. We so appreciate everyone's offers to help, but I really don't know what anyone can do at the moment. There was a Childhood Cancer Rally on the steps of the Capital Building in Washington, D.C. last weekend. I know many from my email group attended. I wish I could harness everyone's willingness to help, and do something that would really make a difference.

Tom and I met with the child psychologist this evening. I'm not sure that we learned anything new, but he did help us find the words to use when talking to the girls. He advised us to be truthful and not "soften" the news. He said that they need to be prepared for what they will be seeing day to day and need time to emotionally prepare for the future. I also asked a few moms in my email group, who have recently lost a child, how they dealt with this issue. They all said the same thing. They were honest with their other children and the sick child just seemed to "know." We plan to tell the girls soon. We have also been perusing the bookstores looking for books that will help all of us cope.

Jonathan had another normal day today. Our sitter, Donna, called this evening and offered Tom and Jonathan their tickets to Thursday night's Red Wings game. Jonathan quickly accepted. Thank you, Donna and Mike. They will have so much fun!

Wednesday, 9/27 ~ Last day of work

I stayed up until 4:00 am last night to complete some last-minute, work-related details to make my leaving a bit easier on others. I met with our Personnel Director and made arrangements to take an indefinite leave of absence. (As I truly enjoy my job, I assured him that I would eventually return.) Jonathan said yesterday that he has never been to Uncle Mike's house, and that he really wants to go. So I spent the rest of the afternoon trying to book flights to Washington, D.C. With all of our canceled and postponed trips to New York, each of us has a number of credits, vouchers, and reimbursements to our name. It was so confusing that the ticket agent asked if I could come in in-person to work through our travel ledger. Four hours later, I owed them $15 for five tickets to Washington, D.C. We are now free and clear of all travel credits. (I do have to say that Northwest Airlines has been very accommodating of our situation!) We plan to leave for DC on Friday morning and return Sunday afternoon.

Thursday, 9/28 ~ Red Wings game and Girls night out

Well, today was my first day as a stay-at-home Mom. Let's see – I overslept, woke the girls up late, realized I don't know how to make school lunches, and sent Elizabeth off to school in a dress on Gym Day. (Melissa says she doesn't know if I'm going to be able to do this!) Jonathan and I took Nana (my Grandma) out to lunch and ran a few errands. Nothing really exciting, but things I don't normally get to do.

Tom, Jonathan, and Grandpa D went to the Red Wings game tonight. They had such a great time! They stopped at Hockeytown for dinner, then learned that someone had arranged for Jonathan to sit in the penalty box during the Red Wings warm-up. One by one, the players skated by and said hello. Darren McCarty and Ken Wreggett gave Jonathan their sticks as they slid into the pen before the start of the game. Jonathan was just in awe! He was then invited to ride on the zamboni while they cleaned the ice between periods, but declined. After the game, Tom, Jonathan, and Grandpa D were escorted into the locker room to meet the players. Tom talked with the players, and McCarty and Wreggett signed their hockey sticks for Jonathan. He came home with a team-autographed stat sheet, the autographed hockey sticks, and his very own Red Wings puck. Jonathan had a wonderful evening, but it is Daddy who is still smiling! I can't believe they forgot to take a camera ... Thanks again, Mike and Donna!

Since Jonathan said they were having a "Boys Night Out," the girls and I had a "Girls Night Out." So instead of a game, we went out to dinner and then went shopping. Over dinner, I decided to take the opportunity to talk to the girls about Jonathan. They knew that Jonathan's cancer was back and that we have been communicating with his doctors. I started by telling them that, although it doesn't look like it, we learned from the doctors that Jonathan is very, very sick. I reminded them that, at the time of Jonathan's diagnosis, we were told that he had a 10-15% chance of getting better. We talked about how well he responded to the initial treatment but how a few of his cancer cells must have survived. I recapped that when we discovered that those cancer cells were continuing to grow, and that there was little that doctors could do here, it was then that we decided to go to New York to try something new. Melissa quickly interjected "but that didn't work either." I then gently explained that there just isn't anything left for the doctors to do, and that Jonathan might start getting even sicker. I then started explaining how people will be stopping by our house periodically to check on Jonathan and to help if we need it, when in the middle of my story, Elizabeth said, "Mom, you're scaring me." Melissa quickly jumped in, "Can we change the subject??" I guess I'm not very good at story-telling! But I continued. I then explained that Jonathan seems to know that he is sick, and that he doesn't seem to be afraid. I was in the middle of telling them that if they were ever sad or if they ever had any questions, they could come to me or Daddy. But in the middle of my story, the girls wanted to go to the bathroom – anything to get away from Mom and the topic at hand! I told them they could go to the bathroom but, while they were away, I wanted each of them to think of a question. And then when they got back, they could each ask their question, I would answer it, and then we would change the subject, and start shopping!

Elizabeth came out of the bathroom and started running across the restaurant. Half way back to the table, she yelled, "I have my question!" As she sat down, she paused, then softly asked, "Mom, do you think Jonathan is going to die?" I fumbled for an answer then told her that there is no cure for Jonathan's cancer and that, yes, he might die. Elizabeth started to cry. And Melissa, who had sat down shortly after

Liz, quietly said that he couldn't die because it would be too quiet at home without Buzz. Then we started talking about all the funny things that Buzz does – like how he hides under the sheets and thinks that no one can see him to how he thinks that taking turns means that he is always first. We agreed that we would not discuss this with Buzz, but that we would try to do many of the things that he likes to do.

The girls decided they wanted to buy Jonathan a present. We went to Toys R Us, and they picked out Gator Golf. (Jonathan saw it on TV and recently added it to his "need" list!) They wrapped it up and it's sitting on the kitchen counter waiting for him to open in the morning. Now that I think about it, we never did get to Melissa's question. We are leaving for Washington D.C. tomorrow morning at 7:30 am.

Saturday, 9/30 ~ Trip cut short

It was sort of a nice trip … We left as scheduled early Friday morning. We got to my brother's house about 2:00 pm. Jonathan was thrilled to see Uncle Mike and loved being at his house. Soon after, we went downtown to the Mall area to do some sightseeing. It was a beautiful day. We video-taped the kids running up and down the steps of the monuments and rolling down the hill of the Jefferson Memorial. We saved the Roosevelt Memorial for last because we wanted to see it at night. We went out for pizza about 9:00 pm and then headed back to the hotel about 10:30 pm to swim. Out of the blue, Jonathan started screaming that his leg hurt. (He generally doesn't do anything quietly!) After trying unsuccessfully to calm him down, I decided to take Jonathan into the hot tub thinking it might make his leg feel better. I got yelled at by the hotel lifeguard (how many hotels have a lifeguard?!?) because they don't allow "children" in the hot tub. I briefly explained his condition and said that I thought the warm water might help his leg. She said, "No problem." I found out later that while we were in the hot tub she called Washington Children's Hospital to make sure that it was ok to take a child with cancer in a hot tub. For some reason, that really annoyed me! Mind your own business!! Anyway, his leg seemed to be bothering him more and more. He ended up screaming and crying off and on throughout the night. At one point when he was crying in the middle of the night, Elizabeth, who snuck a number of stuffed stowaways in her suitcase, got up and gently surrounded him with her large collection of stuffed animals. By early morning, he was screaming, "I want to go to the doc!!!!" Not knowing the area, at 4:00 am, I called my brother and said that we needed to find a hospital. He picked us up and took us to Georgetown University Medical Center. I was nervous about taking Jonathan to a new hospital, but the staff at Georgetown was awesome. I quickly explained our situation and said that we needed something to manage his pain. They quickly gave him a dose of Dilaudid (what we found helpful in New York) and he soon fell asleep. He slept peacefully for about an hour and then woke up complaining that his leg hurt again. After a dose of oral morphine, he fell back to sleep. I then asked the hospital staff for something we could use to manage his pain until we could get back home and set up an appointment with the hospice team. (I guess I should have called them back.) They readily gave us a prescription for oral morphine and a variety of medical supplies to help get us home and through the weekend. We then went to a local drugstore to fill the prescription. After waiting for a very long time, the pharmacist finally came out and said that she couldn't fill the prescription because they didn't have the drug in stock in the same concentration as the written prescription and that federal law prohibits altering the prescription of a narcotic. What?!?! I thought to myself, "I don't need to know all this! I just want some pain med to get us home!!" She then said that we would have to go back to the hospital (a 30-minute drive) and have someone re-write the prescription. Just wanting to get Jonathan back to Michael's, I begged her to call the ER doctor at Georgetown who had written the prescription. Perhaps he could phone it in. Or fax it in. She refused saying she needed a "written" prescription before she could fill it. I was about to blow up when she finally relented and called the hospital. The pharmacist and ER doctor then proceeded to argue on the phone (the ER doctor on our behalf) until the pharmacist eventually backed down and filled the prescription. We finally got back to Michael's, and Jonathan slept most of the afternoon. He seemed to need the pain med, however, about every four hours. We were very nervous about being so far from home, not knowing if this was a fluke or if the pain was going to continue. Tom and I decided to call and reschedule our flights so that we could fly home right away. We gave Jonathan a dose of morphine right before the plane took off and he slept the entire flight. (There were very few people on the flight and Northwest, once again, upgraded our seats to first-class at no extra charge.) Jonathan woke up in the car on the way home from the airport and said that his leg still hurt. We gave him another dose of morphine before he went to bed.

A friend from school gave me a book about a woman who died during surgery and then came back to life. She supposedly remembered much of her journey and transition back. I finished the book during the flight home tonight and am comforted that her journey took her beyond our earthly world. True or not, I am much more at peace after reading the book. Thank you, Rob.

October 2000

Sunday, 10/1 ~ Much, much better today!
Well, I can't believe it. Jonathan slept all night and seemed to be back to normal this morning. While running, however, I did see him stop a few times, grab his leg, and say, "Oooh, my leg!" but then he would quickly resume running and playing. Maybe it was all the hills and stairs, or just too much walking – I don't know. We went to Lynn and Sal's for dinner tonight. Tom's Dad shared some books that he purchased that he thought might be helpful to the kids. We also received word tonight that our neighbors have organized a dinner schedule. That is just so kind ... Thank you, Julie and Kitty.

Monday, 10/2 ~ Still achy
Jonathan got up at 8:00 am this morning and started to get ready for school. School doesn't start until noon, but he wanted me to take him at 9:00 am so he could be first in line. He just loves going to preschool. I talked with his teacher today, and we agreed that I would continue to bring Jonathan to school. I assured her that I would always be close by (most likely in the lobby or parking lot!), and she said she would call if he didn't feel well or wanted to go home. He complained off and on today that his leg, stomach, and/or arm hurt. But he didn't want any medication, and it didn't seem to slow him down. Hospice called back this morning and I reluctantly scheduled our assessment. They

are coming tomorrow at 10:00 am. I guess I do have a lot of questions.

Grandpa D and the SOS Club (Students Offering Services) at Tom's school have been working to arrange a hot air balloon ride for Jonathan. (He still remembers that we took a plane to Florida, not a hot air balloon!) If the winds are calm tomorrow, he and Grandpa are going up!

Tuesday, 10/3 ~ Hospice visit and balloon ride

Hospice came this morning. Grandma D and Grandma E also came for the visit. I was glad to hear that they only work with pediatric patients. The hospice team talked at length about all the services they can provide and what we should expect in the coming weeks/months. The two women were very forthright in their explanations, and the conversation was difficult at times. But don't get me wrong – that is what I want! It was hard to concentrate on the topic at hand, however, with Jonathan kicking a football around the back yard wearing oversized sunglasses and a cool-looking Hawaiian shirt. They said that the good days/bad days that we have been experiencing are not uncommon at this point. They explained that a patient might have a bad day (like Saturday in Washington, D.C.) buried amongst a number of good days. But over time, the number of good days will decrease as the number of bad days increases, until eventually, the bad days will greatly outnumber the good. Right now, I'm not sure how I feel about hospice. I know that we will need their services – especially for pain management – but I'm not ready to relinquish control.

Yay, for light winds!! Jonathan and Grandpa D finally got their balloon ride! (Because there was extra room in the balloon, Daddy and Liz also got to hop in at the last minute.) Elizabeth and Jonathan were so excited. As the balloon lifted higher and higher, Jonathan yelled, "Bye Momma! ... I love you! ... I gonna mit you!" Grandma D, Grandma E, Melissa, and I followed the balloon in the van. After struggling to find a place to land, they gently crashed down at dusk in a small, open field. We then went back and had dinner with the Balloon Man at a local restaurant. We got a lot of great pictures and video clips!

Wednesday, 10/4 ~ Another bad night

Jonathan woke up about midnight last night crying that his arm hurt. You can just tell that it is not a "normal" ache or pain. We gave him a dose of morphine and he fell asleep about 15-20 minutes later. He then slept straight through until 11:30 am this morning.

I was just kind of sad this morning. After I got the girls off to school, I climbed back in bed with Jonathan and fell asleep next to him. (He doesn't know it, but he missed school today because we slept so long.) The first thing he said when he woke up was that his arm hurt. A few hours later, he accepted three Children's Tylenols (his bubble gum meds). He complained off and on throughout the day that his body hurt, but didn't want any more med.

Jonathan and I went out this afternoon to buy pumpkins and some Halloween decorations at a local farm. I planned on buying three pumpkins, one for each kid, but came home with eight (one's even a little mushy!) because Jonathan just couldn't leave his new painted "friends" behind. I'm not very good at saying "no" right now.

Friday, 10/6 ~ Jonathan's idea

We decided to monitor Jonathan's pain medication a bit more closely. The hospice nurse suggested we be a bit proactive, rather than reactive, by giving Jonathan a small dose of med every 4-5 hours to hopefully prevent the breakthrough pain. His arm really seems to be bothering him. We tried the periodic smaller doses all last night and all day today, and it seems to be helping.

Jonathan was very excited about school today because it was his turn to be the "leader." When you are the leader, it is your turn for show-and-tell, and you get to bring the snack for the class. (Get to bring the snack ... his teacher is so smart!!) He did not want to miss being the leader! I could tell his arm was bothering him as we walked into school, and I asked him if he wanted to go back home. He said, "No. But I have a 'dea. How 'bout if you go home and get me some med and then come right back?!" So Mom went home, got the med, and then stayed at school with him for the rest of the day. (Now I know why I don't teach preschool!!) He also started complaining of a headache this afternoon. I stayed up late last night and read about 20-25 children's books dealing with death, dying, and grief. I'm trying to find some good ones for the kids.

Sunday, 10/8 ~ Honest feelings

Jonathan complained of a headache all weekend. Yesterday, he was sooo cranky—yelling, screaming, arguing with the girls, etc. He finally said he is tired of his arm hurting and his head aching. He just wants to be Buzz.

Jonathan spent last night at Grandma and Grandpa D's with cousins, Zach and Anna, while Melissa and Elizabeth spent the night at Grandma and Grandpa E.'s. Tom and I just needed a night to vent about all that we have been feeling. We ended up going out to dinner with Chris, Laurie, and Laura. (Tim was out of town.) It was nice to get out and have a chance to talk openly with adults. I shared that I have been increasingly overwhelmed by everything that is going on and feel like I am the only one who is "worrying" about everything. Others pointed out that Tom and I are reacting with classic "Tom" and "Rhonda" personalities. The best analogy is going back to school in September. Once the calendar says August 1st, I start thinking about school, talking about school, and preparing for school. I have to do this in order to be physically ready and mentally prepared for the first day of school. Tom says I waste my last three weeks of summer "worrying" about the first day. Tom doesn't want to think about school or talk about school until the day before. Then it slaps him in the face and he accepts that school has begun. We realized that we are dealing with Jonathan's illness the same way. I want to research everything, know everything, and be fully prepared for what is to come. Tom just wants to enjoy the time we have. It helps to know that we have both accepted the reality but just deal with it differently day to day. We agreed that I would try to spend more time enjoying the present and that Tom would slowly acclimate himself to making some future plans. I plan to visit some funeral homes and cemeteries on Thursday. Tom said he is not ready for this (and I am certainly not going alone!) so I begged my sister Laurie to accompany me.

Melissa, Elizabeth, and Jonathan spent Sunday afternoon with Uncle Dan and Aunt Nic. Dan and Nicole entertained the kids with craft projects and games. We then had the family over for dinner. After dinner, as the cousins played, the adults spent some time flipping through the pile of children's books. Grandma D got Melissa to read one of the books with her. Soon after, as we were tucking the girls in bed, Melissa asked if I would lay with her. Moments later, she just melted down and started bawling. She said she just wants to be a normal family like all of her friends. After a good, long cry and some open, honest words, I think she felt a little bit better. Melissa then pulled out one of her beanie babies and said, "This one always reminds me of Buzz." She then carefully chose four more until she had recreated our whole family. She fell asleep holding the beanie family of five.

Monday, 10/9 ~ Sleeping late
Jonathan slept until 1:00 pm today. When he woke up, he was in exceptionally great spirits. He said he had a "really good dream" last night, but that he didn't remember what it was about.

He has been very restless at night—tossing, turning, talking out loud, etc. We are going to start giving him more Tylenol to see if that helps ease the headaches. He was disappointed to learn that he slept through school again today. Elizabeth's teacher stopped by this afternoon. We had a really nice visit. It is reassuring to know that girls' teachers are watching over them. Thank you, Debbie. Right now, Jonathan is at a basketball game with Tom and Melissa.

Tuesday, 10/10 ~ No news is good news
Jonathan got up at 8:00 am today because he didn't want to miss another day of school. He was disappointed again when I told him that today wasn't a school day. Donna, our

sitter, came over today so I could run some errands. I felt so guilty not spending this beautiful day with Jonathan that I could not think straight or enjoy my time alone. I came home after a few hours with little accomplished. Jonathan, however, enjoyed his day with Ms. Donna, probably because she lets him win when they play cards. Jonathan took an afternoon nap but seemed to feel pretty good today.

Wednesday, 10/11 ~ Black eye is back

Jonathan slept in again – this time until 12:00 pm. I thought about waking him up earlier but noticed that his eye was black again and looked rather swollen. I decided to let him sleep. He also complained of headaches throughout the day. The hospice nurse was supposed to come today but called and postponed her visit until Friday. I am going to call the doctor tomorrow to see if we should pursue some radiation to his eye. My guess is that the headaches are related to the black eye. Jonathan spent most of the day lying on the couch watching cartoons.

Thursday, 10/12 ~ Gathering info

Laurie and I spent the afternoon visiting funeral homes and cemeteries. There are just too many decisions to make to save everything to the last minute. Part of me wants to start discussing these things now while another part of me doesn't want to spend any time away from Jonathan working on such details. Now I know why people just pick "a package deal." But I can't do that. Jonathan is too special. We also discovered that the selection of caskets for children is minimal. (Basic law of supply and demand.) So far, nothing is acceptable in my book. We are going to have a traditional funeral, but the biggest decision we have to make is whether to have him buried or cremated. I kind of want to have him buried so that we have a place to visit, but I also know that Jonathan is afraid of the dark and doesn't like to sleep alone. I worry that I would not be able to sleep at night thinking of him ... out there ... all by himself. Tom and I haven't talked much about this yet as we are rarely alone. I also haven't had a chance to share with him what Laurie and I learned today.

We have an appointment with the radiologist tomorrow afternoon. Jonathan's eye is now very black, slightly swollen, and bloodshot in the corner. I am hoping we can radiate the site. We cancelled the visit with the hospice nurse as it conflicted with the radiology appointment. We will reschedule sometime next week. We have cut back on the pain meds, and he seems to be doing ok.

Friday, 10/13 ~ A really bad headache
Jonathan woke up early today and said that he had a "really, really, really bad headache." He complained that his head hurt for most of the day. Tom took Jonathan to the radiologist this afternoon. Dr. Chuba thinks he can radiate his eye and his arm with little or no side effects. He thinks the eye can return to normal and that the radiation might help relieve his arm pain. We are going to start the prep work next Wednesday and begin radiating the following Monday. I don't like waiting a week and a half before doing something to his eye. He says it doesn't bother him, but it is really starting to look bad. Grandma Jo (Tom's Grandma) came by for lunch today, and because Jonathan missed multiple days of school, his teacher dropped by with the art projects from the past week. She said the kids at school are asking about Jonathan. We agreed that I would write a letter to all the parents and that she would discuss Jonathan's illness

with his classmates. His preschool teacher, Mrs. T, is just awesome. We visited with friends, Janet and Ryan, and the Ferraris this evening. Janet and Ryan brought their dog. The kids had a ball! I think Elizabeth needs a pet ...

Saturday, 10/14 ~ Ref says "time-out!

Elizabeth spent the night at my sister's last night and Michelle, Melissa's best friend, spent the night at our house. Jonathan slept between Melissa and Michelle in the pup tent that the girls put up in Melissa's room. Melissa and Michelle's teacher, Mr. Stuehmer, came over to meet Jonathan and to play basketball with the girls. He said Melissa talks about Jonathan a lot at school. Mr. Stuehmer and the neighborhood kids played basketball on Michelle's driveway while Jonathan played referee. He loves to blow his whistle and call time-outs! Later in the day Melissa asked, "Mom? What wrong with Jonathan's eye?" She said she didn't notice it before now (or perhaps chose to ignore it).

Later we went to Anna's birthday party and then to an apple orchard/petting farm. Jonathan asked for very little med today. I think the day was full of fun-filled "distractions." Ironically, Mom is very worn down and probably needs some med.

Monday, 10/16 ~ Now his leg hurts

Last night, Jonathan started complaining that his leg hurt again – probably from having too much fun yesterday. This morning he was kind of limping around. He still wanted to go to school though and is very excited about his upcoming field trip to the apple orchard on Wednesday. I was worried about how his classmates would react when they saw his black eye. His teacher said that no one even seemed to notice. (Kids don't get all stressed out about things, do they??) We postponed the radiation simulation until next Tuesday so that Jonathan won't miss the field trip to the apple orchard. He keeps talking about the last field trip in which his classmates "went without me." Hopefully, we can begin the radiation treatments within a day or so after the simulation.

Tuesday, 10/17 ~ A bad day

No ... it was an awful day. In summary, Jonathan felt really sick, the girls had an emotional breakdown, and Mom, who has a severe cold, needs to go to bed. More details tomorrow.

Wednesday, 10/18 ~ Emotions ramping up

First of all, about yesterday ... Jonathan has not been sleeping well. He wants me to be right next to him with my arm around him and his arm around me. I love sleeping with him, but if I try to move my arm, he wakes up and says, "Snug me, Momma!" He also seemed to have a fever off and on throughout the night. Needless to say, I also didn't sleep very well. Then he woke up yesterday morning unable to walk. He tried to walk a few times, but his legs just shook and he was unable to support himself. He just looked at me with big, sad eyes. I just melted down inside. I carried him to the couch, and we watched cartoons ... lots and lots of cartoons. He didn't want to leave the couch, and he wanted me to hold him the entire time. He seemed very uncomfortable and kept asking for more med. I kept trying different things, but he just wasn't comfortable. After five hours of mindless cartoons, (although I kind of liked CatDog, especially when Jonathan said, "You be cat and I'll be dog"), he finally fell asleep. He woke up later and wanted more med. He also hadn't eaten anything all day. By 8:00 pm, he wanted some dry cereal and a glass of milk. As soon as he finished, he yelled that he was going to throw up. The girls were upstairs in their bedrooms, and they heard him getting sick. Elizabeth immediately started screaming and crying which prompted Melissa to start yelling at her. Melissa screamed, "Stop it! You don't know how it feels to have cancer!!" Elizabeth continued to scream, Melissa started crying, and I was stuck holding a bucket next to Jonathan.

Tom quickly came up from the basement and ran upstairs to calm the girls. They soon stopped screaming and crying, and Jonathan said he felt better after throwing up. We then went upstairs to talk with the girls. Elizabeth confided that she is afraid that Jonathan might die at any minute. She said kids at school keep asking her "if her brother died yet." She wants me to come in to her 3rd grade classroom and talk with her classmates. And she wants Buzz to sit on her lap while I am there. (At least she can clearly articulate what she wants!) Melissa said she updates her class everyday about Buzz during "circle time." (Melissa happened to see this online Journal yesterday and, on her own, signed the Guestbook. I'm not sure how much she read.) So I asked the girls if they would like to read a few more of Mom's special books. We chose one about two little girls whose little brother dies. Bad choice – too close to home. Elizabeth started crying when I flipped open the cover, and I was crying by page two. Melissa grabbed the book from me and said, "Then I'll read the book." She got me and Elizabeth a tissue, and then read the book aloud. At the end of the story, we talked about the two little girls. One of the girls in the story was very sad and cried a lot. Elizabeth said, "That's like me." The other girl was also sad but kept many of her feelings to herself. Melissa said, "That's more like me." Elizabeth felt better when we told her that the doctors and nurses would tell us when Buzz was really, really, really sick and that for now, she should just play with him like always. Jonathan never did eat anything all day and never left the couch.

Also, out of the blue yesterday, Jonathan said that he wanted to tell everyone that he believes in Jesus. But he couldn't do it from home; he needed to be in church. I'm not sure quite how to say this, but I don't know where this is all coming from. We just recently started attending church, and Tom and I are still working on finding our own personal faith. The kids seem to enjoy church, but they certainly haven't been exposed to religion and Bible stories at home. And furthermore, Jonathan spends most of his time in church lying on the floor drawing pictures and eating Cheerios! As soon as Jonathan woke up this morning, however, he reminded me that he needed to go to church.

Jonathan woke up looking and feeling a bit better this morning. He still couldn't walk though and had trouble rolling over in bed. But today he had things he wanted to do. Grandma and Grandpa E came for a visit, and we had to carry him up and down the stairs, and around the house, gathering all of his important things. By lunchtime, he seemed to be doing a bit better. He took a few steps here and there but was still moving slowly. We then went to Toys R Us because he decided he needed a panda bear like one of his cartoon friends. Of course, Toys R Us didn't have any panda bears, and he was smart enough to know that the brown bear that Mom was pushing was not a panda bear. By the time we got home, he seemed to be feeling much better and was walking almost like normal. Grandma and Grandpa D and the Frontieros came by this evening.

I am starting to feel very overwhelmed. Every day is so unpredictable, and I am not good at that. I need a quiet day at home without a "crisis," without the phone ringing, without commotion, just a day to relax. If you get my answering machine tomorrow, please don't take it personally ...

Thursday, 10/19 ~ A quiet day

Wow – only two phone calls today. Maybe more people read this than I realize. Thanks for the break.

The soap opera, however, continues. Last night, Melissa woke up feeling sick at 4:00 am. At 6:00 am, Elizabeth woke up not feeling well. I finally got everyone back to sleep by 7:00 am, turned off the alarm for school, and decided that we could all use a day to sleep in. But today, Jonathan woke up at 8:30 am, nice and peppy!! He then proceeded to wake everyone else up. Melissa flipped out when she realized that she was missing school and insisted that I drive her right away. (She was sitting in the back seat of the car with her backpack when I was still in my nightgown. She cracks me up!) Elizabeth, whose favorite subject is recess, decided that she needed to stay home. It was a selfish decision on my part, but Elizabeth and Jonathan played together all day, and it gave me a much needed break. Jonathan had good and bad moments throughout the day. He's still walking a bit tentatively and wants to be carried up and down the stairs. But if you don't act fast enough, and he really wants something, he can still do it on his own. The hospice team also stopped by for a short visit this afternoon.

Monday, 10/23 ~ Very cranky!
Jonathan has not been himself lately. Although he has not complained about pain for several days now, he has been incredibly cranky—screaming, crying, throwing tantrums, etc. I am sure there is more going on "behind the scenes." I have no idea how a four-year-old deals with knowing he has cancer, knowing he might die, not feeling well, wanting med, not liking to take med, wanting to play, feeling like he can't play, etc. I'm not quite sure how to help him …

Pastor Jon stopped by Friday afternoon, but Jonathan wasn't up for visiting. Tom and Grandpa D took Elizabeth and Jonathan to the Michigan/Michigan State football game Saturday afternoon, and we attended cousins Jessica and Samantha's baptism yesterday. While shopping for the girls' baptism gifts, we picked out a few Bible stories for part of their gift. With all that's been happening, I wanted the books to be from Jonathan. So I asked Jonathan what he would he like to say to his cousins. After thinking for a moment, he answered, "Just tell them 'Jesus will take care of you.'" I inscribed the books with his words, and he signed his name. His message was very short, very reassuring, and very sincere.

We also noticed a new tumor on the side of his cheek near his ear. It is very round, about the size of a marble. He is scheduled for a CT scan tomorrow.

Tuesday, 10/24 ~ Much more content!
Jonathan was in a great mood all day yesterday and this morning. Last night we played his favorite songs and

danced around the living room. He wrestled, tackled, twisted, turned, and chattered away. He was good, old, "normal" Buzz. I couldn't stop squeezing him. But it was short-lived. About 1:30 this afternoon, he started screaming and crying that his arm hurt. He either has a new tumor on his arm or a big, swollen mosquito bite. (It might sound silly, but they look the same.) Regardless, we are back to pain med. It seemed to take a few hours before we got the pain under control. He finally fell asleep about 8:30 pm.

I seem to be having a hard time remembering things and keeping up with everyday life. Yesterday, I found a cereal box in the refrigerator. The girls' backpacks and school papers – I've given up trying to keep them organized. And then today, Jonathan and I went to the hospital for the CT scan. We got there at 10:30 am, but discovered that we were supposed to be there for a simulation appointment at 8:30 am. I don't know how I missed that part!! And they couldn't do the CT scan without doing the simulation first, so now we have to go back tomorrow at 3:00 pm for the simulation and scan. I just want to know about all these new lumps ... now! On the other hand, Jonathan told me today that I was the "bestest Mom." So, ha! Beat that!! I guess that's all that really matters. I have been sorting pictures. I discovered that I have hundreds of pictures (literally) of Melissa, our first baby, and maybe ten of Jonathan. Guess I'm not the fairest Mom ...

Wednesday, 10/25 ~ Mixed messages
Jonathan and I spent the afternoon at St. John Hospital. We had the simulation and CT scan done. Dr. Chuba thinks the new lump near his ear is a diseased lymph node. If so, that means that the disease has progressed to his lymphatic

system and is most likely growing in other nodes as well. At the same time, he thinks he can manage most of Jonathan's pain right now through radiation. We are going to radiate his eye, lymph node, arm and hip area. When Dr. Chuba saw Jonathan crying about his arm hurting today, he said he would fit him in right away. So tomorrow we are starting arm radiation and will then complete the simulation on his leg. Radiation at the other sites will follow within days.

Dr. Chuba seems very optimistic. He told me about a pediatric oncology conference he recently attended in Amsterdam, Germany. While there, he met a neuroblastoma researcher who is working on a new radioactive treatment protocol. He discussed Jonathan's case with the researcher and is going to make some calls on our behalf. We are just so grateful and so amazed by all that the hospital staff is doing to help. We should get the CT results back tomorrow. I'm curious if the disease shows up anywhere else in his head ...

Friday, 10/27 ~ Good news and bad news ...

Well, good news and bad news. The CT scan shows no evidence of cancer in Jonathan's brain, but today, Laurie noticed two small, new lumps on his chest while we were helping him get dressed. (We only did a CT scan of his head). He has now had two days of radiation. We have a standing daily appointment, and he is on the table for less than 10 minutes. He didn't like getting his tattoo marks (laser guidelines) but now proudly shows them to everyone. Tom and I are having second thoughts on all the radiation and feel we need to better clarify our goals. It seems futile to radiate every new spot that appears; that's just a game we will not win. So right now we have decided to focus on just two spots – his arm to minimize the pain and his eye for cosmetic reasons. We are noticing that even the medical professionals don't agree on what is the best course of action at this time. We are frustrated that we have no one professional to turn to for guidance. That said, we made the executive decision to cancel radiation on Tuesday because going Trick-or-Treating is much more important at the moment!

Saturday, 10/28 ~ Feeling better

Well, the radiation seems to be working. Jonathan's upper arm is still slightly swollen, but he didn't complain about his arm hurting today. (Although now he says his eye hurts.) Right now, he is playing like normal and back to acting silly.

Tonight was fun! We invited the family over for a Halloween Party. The kids carved pumpkins, bobbed for apples, and played games in the basement. Jonathan even took a turn whacking the piñata. The holidays, however, are stressing me out. I can't stop thinking that each one might be his last. Jonathan is dressing up as Tigger this year. He said he wants to be Pikachu next year. Right now, he is in a Winnie-the-Pooh phase. We also had to buy a jar of honey at the grocery store today so that Jonathan could eat honey just like Pooh. Tomorrow is Jonathan's big day at church.

Sunday, 10/29 ~ Whole-church prayer

Wow! What an awesome experience. In Melissa's words, "Jonathan got his very own prayer today." Pastor Jon has been so helpful through this whole experience. This morning, he led the entire congregation in a special prayer for Jonathan. Pastor Jon had the entire congregation form concentric circles around Jonathan, With everyone's hand on the shoulder of the person in front of them, all touching Jonathan in the middle, it was an extremely powerful moment. Pastor Jon then gave us the microphone as Jonathan planned to tell everyone at church that "he believes in Jesus." Jonathan got nervous at the last minute, however, and made me do it for him. I took the microphone and told everyone that Jonathan really wanted to come to church today because he had something he wanted to say. With Jonathan looking somberly at the floor, I told everyone that Jonathan wanted them to know that he believes in Jesus. I then went on to explain that something very real and very incredible seemed to be happening. Jonathan, on his own, felt it important to make this public affirmation. Pastor Jon then gave Jonathan two Bibles – one from Shepherd's Gate and the other a Children's Bible of his very own. Jonathan seems to be at peace when he is at church. And Melissa and Elizabeth were touched that so many people cared so much about their little brother. Tom and I are still a bit in awe of all that is happening …

Oh, and Jonathan said he doesn't like honey, unlike Pooh.

Monday, 10/30 ~ Visit to school

Tom, Jonathan, and I visited Elizabeth's third grade classroom today. (Tom was one of the Pumpkin Dads!) Elizabeth wanted her classmates to see that Jonathan is ok. While I was there, I heard a few remarks from her classmates that I know would make Elizabeth uncomfortable. One little girl went up to Jonathan and started teasing him about having cancer. He just sat quietly in his chair. We talked about the incident on the way home. I told him if anyone ever said something like that to him again, that he could bop 'em!!

Jonathan laughed! (Sorry, I will try to act like an adult.) But it was a successful visit. The class (and Jonathan) also seemed to enjoy the Pumpkin Math activity. While at school, we also stopped in Melissa's 5th grade classroom. Melissa's classmates treated Buzz like he was their class mascot. He joined circle time and enjoyed entertaining the class.

Jonathan and I went to radiation again this afternoon. Since the radiation seems to be minimizing the pain, we added a few more sites. We are now radiating his arm, eye, leg, and hip. The actual radiation runs about 30-40 seconds per site. With camera and position changes, he is on the table about 15-20 minutes each day. And he lies perfectly still ... with Mickey, Grover, and vee-vee waiting patiently at the end of the table. I am sure he accepts the radiation mask only because it makes him look like a goalie!

Tuesday, 10/31 ~ Happy Halloween
It's funny how silly, little holidays like Halloween are a BIG deal when your kid has cancer. I don't think Jonathan was feeling very well today but he was so excited about Halloween, it didn't seem to matter. Melissa dressed up as a doctor (who is going to find a cure for cancer), Elizabeth was a witch, and Jonathan was Tigger because "he likes to bounce a lot." The surprise came when Jonathan accidentally stepped on his costume while getting dressed and discovered that his Tigger costume talked! After that, he didn't want or need any candy. He just wanted to make Tigger sounds. Grandma and Grandpa D and Uncle Dan came over for trick-or-treating, and Aunt Joann manned the door. The girls made it around the subdivision while Jonathan lasted about ten houses before getting tired. For some reason, the kids received an excessive amount of candy this

year. Best of all, we just had fun!! Buzz says, "Happy Birthday, Uncle Mike!!'"

November 2000

Wednesday, 11/1 ~ Buzz is back!

November – Wow! Every milestone makes me smile, even if it's just a month. Speaking of smiling, Jonathan smiled all through radiation today. He complained earlier this morning that he didn't want to go to radiation because "the mask is too tight." So I told him they just needed to get a couple of good "pictures" and then we'd be out of there! So during radiation – in the room all by himself – he had the biggest grin on his face. He wanted those pictures to turn out great so we could blow that popsicle stand!! One of the nurses gave our name to another mom whose child was recently diagnosed with cancer. We met for coffee today in the hospital cafe.

Best news of all – Buzz's personality is back!! He seems to be feeling great today and hasn't complained of pain for days. It feels like a plateau. He was full of energy and bounce today, just like normal. He said his sweatshirt got stuck on his head because he had really big brains. He taunted Elizabeth with "finda keepa; losa weepa (finders, keepers; losers, weepers). He went "swimming" in the Jacuzzi bathtub wearing his plastic safety goggles. He said he beat Ms. Donna in Go Fish and Old Maid "without even cheating!" He watched Melissa's basketball game through Happy Meal binoculars. And he climbed up onto our bed all by himself for the first time in weeks! He was loud and silly, and he chattered and teased all day long. Tom and I just keep looking at each other and smiling! Our Buzz is back!

Friday, 11/3 ~ Oral chemo?

We had radiation bright and early today. Each treatment is making his eye look better. We have eight more sessions to go. Jonathan felt great today and spent most the day waiting for Daddy to get home from school so that they could play hockey. (Mom tried but he told me I wasn't very good.) Dr. Sawaf called today to ask how Jonathan was doing. We so appreciated his call. I discussed with him the conflicting opinions we have been getting and how difficult it is to make decisions with little or no medical "data." We also discussed giving Jonathan some oral chemotherapy. Because he is doing so well right now, we are looking for ways to maximize his quality time. On the other hand, we do not want these "good" days to be filled with anxiety and tension about having to drink "the yucky med." Dr. Chuba proposed giving Jonathan the chemo and watching the external tumors. If they continue to grow, then we will know the chemo is not working and can stop treatment. If they start to shrink, however, we can surmise that the chemo is helping and that it might help slow the progression of disease. If Jonathan is willing to drink the chemo, we agreed to start tomorrow. And just when I think I can breathe again … Tom picked Jonathan up tonight and felt a new lump (a big one) under his arm. I'm guessing another lymph node. Now I'm stressed again and don't know if we should start the chemo or not. Back to square one.

Earlier this evening, Jonathan and I were lying in bed. As I held him, my eyes filled with tears. "What's wrong's, Momma?" I didn't know quite what to say, but said through my tears, "I'm just mad at God for giving you cancer." Jonathan then shot back matter-of-factly, "God didn't give me cancer. It just came to me." After a short pause, he added, "We're not taking very good care of our Earth, you know." He continues to amaze me ...

Monday, 11/6 ~ Started oral chemo

We had a normal (busy) weekend. Jonathan is still doing great, but ... I think I am starting to fall apart. Even Tom has noticed. I am filled with stress and anxiety. I just cannot shake the thoughts that consume me all day long. I am getting annoyed with my own attitude. We decided to start the chemo on the premise that we have nothing to lose, and perhaps some quality time to gain.

Jonathan also found the Christmas ornaments in the basement today and wants it to be Christmas. We're going to put our tree and lights up this weekend. Our neighbors are going to think we're a bit overzealous.

Friday, 11/10 ~ Mom's secret

Wow, it's been four days since I updated. So, I've been trying to get Tom to write an entry, but so far, no dice. But, guess what? I found out today that he logs in everyday to read my posts!! That's ok. He doesn't mop the kitchen floor either. (Ok, in the interest of full disclosure, he does do a lot of other things.) I also needed a few days to think about how much I wanted to share.

Jonathan has been doing really well. He has been running around, playing hockey, teasing the girls, etc. It's ironic, but since he's been feeling better, I've been feeling worse. This slight reprieve has given me a chance to realize how sad, uptight, and emotional I've become. I was reading the other night that you can begin grieving for someone before they die. (I didn't know that.) I fit the description to a tee. I just want to sit and hold Jonathan. Anyway—I'm not sure if I want everyone to know this, but in the interest of other cancer moms—I have started taking a mild antidepressant, anti-anxiety medication. I don't like this—I hate taking medication—but I'm tired of feeling down and stressed. The doctor described my condition as "situational anxiety and depression." Situational anxiety and depression is supposed to go away on its own after the "situation" has resolved itself. My concern is that the situation is not going to "resolve itself;" it is just going to get worse! I am worried that I will forever be different and need to find some way to work through this on my own. It is changing who I am and my outlook on life. I'll let you know if the med works ...

We have four more days of radiation. Jonathan's eye, however, is looking a little blacker today, and he complained of a headache earlier this morning. (But he also told me that he gets a headache if he watches cartoons all day. Yeah, right—Mom too!) He also has three new toys on his wish list—fresh from those cartoon TV commercials—so we are planning to stop at Toys R Us on the way home from the doc. I really don't know what I'd buy this kid for Christmas. He has no wants. ... And that's just the way I want it.

Monday, 11/13 ~ Frazzled nerves
We had a normal weekend—nothing special. Tom worked on the basement, and we had the family over for dinner Sunday night. Jonathan seemed to be his normal self. Our "normal" weekend, however, was broken today on the way to the hospital for radiation. I usually take Jonathan to his radiation appointments by myself. Luckily, my parents were with me today. (Jonathan wanted them to see his "hockey

mask" — his radiation mask.) I was driving and Jonathan was sitting in the backseat with Grandma. About 30 minutes from the hospital, Jonathan started screaming, "My nose! My nose!!" He was bleeding from his nose. Being that he was frightened, he then started yelling, screaming, and jumping around — all of course, making the problem even worse. I pulled over, and Grandma E and I traded places. Jonathan kept screaming that he needed the doc and yelling to Grandma to drive faster. At one point, he said he wished he was in Grandpa D's car because "he drives really fast, like a motorcycle." The bleeding eventually subsided, and we soon arrived at the hospital. Jonathan is generally most comfortable being at the hospital when he has a problem, but he was now afraid to wear the radiation mask. He kept crying that he couldn't wear his mask because his red stuff might start coming out again. We sat in the waiting room, playing games and working puzzles, for about 45 minutes until he calmed down. During that time, he did experience a few more minor nosebleeds. I told him that he didn't have to get his "picture taken" if he didn't want to, but then I worried that if the nosebleeds were due to the tumor pressing on his nasal cavity, that radiation was the only way to reduce or minimize the pressure. We finally bartered that we would let the radiation team take only one picture. We would do the eye (with the mask) when his nose was ok but would not let them do the arm and leg. He liked feeling like he had some control. We got the eye done, but he was uptight the rest of the night about his nose. Mom pretended not to be.

Tuesday, 11/14 ~ Another nosebleed
This is not how I wanted to start my day! Jonathan has not been sleeping well the past few nights. He's been very rest-

less and has been waking up several times during the night. To make things worse, he also seems to have some sort of cold. He woke up about 6:00 am this morning and couldn't breathe due to his cold. I tried to talk him into some kind of cold medicine, but he didn't want to take anything. He continued to sniff and try to breathe until I decided that he had to take something. I got up and offered him two choices: chewable tablets or a liquid medicine. When he wouldn't choose, I made the choice. When he saw me walk into the room with the liquid cold medicine in a cup he started throwing a fit – yelling, screaming (yea, he does that a lot!!), and jumping up and down on the bed. Next thing I know, he is covered in blood. Yep. And so is our bed. He got another nosebleed. Of course, this one coincided with the girls' alarm clock going off so they came down in the middle of this escapade. I somehow got the girls ready for school as I carried Jonathan around and held a washcloth to his nose. I was trying to stay calm in front of the girls, but I was really worried about the nosebleed. His nose had been bleeding for close to an hour now, and I couldn't get it to stop. It would slow down every now and then, but would then resume. I finally got the girls out the door and called my mom for help. By the time my mom got here, Jonathan had fallen asleep with the washcloth on his face. While he slept, I called the hospice nurse. She assured me that if his blood counts were ok, the bleeding would eventually stop. But I did ask, "What if his counts are not ok, and it doesn't stop? Then, what do I do??" She said to take him to the ER. His nose finally stopped bleeding after about two hours, but by then I was a nervous wreck. It's hard to distinguish the fine line between wanting to provide palliative care at home and needing emergency help. I spent the rest of the day with Jonathan on my lap. He told me that I was supposed to sit and watch his nose so that he could watch cartoons. He would sniff and then panic that his nose was going to start to bleed. I had to reassure him that I was watching. He spent the day watching cartoons; I spent the day worrying. By the end of the day, I was not only worried, but equally frustrated.

Everyone keeps telling us that we are in control and that we "get" to make all the decisions. Using the example of Jonathan's nosebleeds, we have expressed our concern about the nosebleeds to many, but no one – except for me – is trying to determine "why" his nose is bleeding. My premise is if we know what is causing the problem, we can better choose an appropriate response. If the nosebleeds are due to the eye tumor, then let's continue the radiation. If the nosebleeds are due to a cold, then let's add some cold medicine. If the nosebleeds are due to low platelets, then let's look into a transfusion. That sounds simple enough, but that isn't happening. There is no cause and effect. It is "just deal with the problems as they appear." For the first time, Tom and I also disagree about what we should be doing. I have backed off on the oral chemo because Jonathan is putting up such a fuss about taking it. If it causes him anxiety every day, I have decided it isn't worth it. To Tom, it is. The real issue is that Tom and I shouldn't be disagreeing about what to do without any data to help guide us. A medical doctor would assess the current situation and make an educated decision. We are being asked to make decisions, about our own child no less, without an accurate assessment. To compound the situation, those involved in his care are giving us conflicting advice. I am greatly annoyed that the tests and diagnostic tools available during active treatment are not routinely used at this stage of the game. While still agreeing to palliative care, I think periodic testing could help us make better educated decisions and help ensure that we have no regrets.

Hospice called this afternoon to see how Jonathan was doing. They probably wish they hadn't called today.

Wednesday, 11/15 ~ Something's not right

Well, after 19 days of no pain meds, Jonathan woke up twice last night complaining that his leg hurt. We gave him a dose of morphine at midnight and then another at 4:00 am. He also complained of a headache a few times this afternoon and accepted some of his bubble gum meds (Tylenols). He had another half dozen nosebleeds today— none of them like yesterday—and spent most of the day sleeping. He was very lethargic and really hasn't eaten much the last few days. The hospice team came by this afternoon and also noticed that he looks very pale. They noted that all of the above are classic symptoms of low blood counts and suggested that we get his counts checked. I don't know if they would have suggested this anyway or if they did so because they know that's what we want to do. Regardless, I am going to pursue this tomorrow. Jonathan was definitely not himself today, although he did manage to call me a "Mutt-yo Head." That's his new word when he's trying to be silly.

Sunday, 11/19 ~ Something is going on …

I've been trying to update for days now. It seems that when I have the most to say, I have the least time. Something is happening. We had a blood draw Thursday afternoon and learned that Jonathan's blood cell counts were extremely low. His hemoglobin was 3.8. Normal is 11-15. His doctor

said that a count of 1-1.5 could cause him to slip into a
coma. So we know that his bone marrow is no longer
producing the necessary blood products. To sustain him,
he will now need blood transfusions. Tom and Jonathan
spent Thursday night in the hospital. Jonathan received a
red blood cell and platelet transfusion. Wow! Night and day!
Jonathan came home Friday morning with lots of energy
and was his chipper self! He called me on the cell phone
on the way home from the hospital and said, "Hi Momma.
We coming home now! I mit you!!" When he got home, he
ran through the house yelling for Bit and Ra-Ra (his name
for Elizabeth and Melissa). What a difference a few cells
can make!!

But his chipper mood was short-lived. By mid-afternoon
he was stressed and filled with anxiety. He oscillated between being tired and overwhelmed, to having a lot of
things that he wanted to do. It was an unbelievable, emotionally demanding day. The shift in demeanor started when
he casually said, "I might die you know" – kind of like he
was warning me about the future and also letting me know
that he had a lot of things to do before that happened.
Then he was so dramatic – crying, with his hands on his
head in agony – "Ooooh, look at Mickey. He has spots on
him! And look at vee-vee!! I need my stuff to be clean!!!"
(He likes everything to be neat, clean, and organized.) He
insisted that I wash Mickey and vee-vee, and the other
Mickey blanket on his bed. I was paranoid at the thought
of washing Mickey, but Jonathan was adamant. As I
dropped Mickey into the washer I was thinking … "Well,
I suppose I could call Disney World and have them Fed-Ex
me another one." I think I opened the lid of the washer
and dryer ten times each to check on poor Mick!!! But he

survived and everything is sparkling clean!! Then, he went up to his room and cried out again with much drama, "Oooohhhh!! Look at my rooooomm!! Now I have to clean this aaalllll up!!" (Jonathan doesn't mess up his room. It gets messed up when friends and cousins visit.) I told him I would help him clean his room. I could tell that it was going to take a very long time. Everything had to be perfect: books lined up, puzzles stacked. Red legos on the left, blue ones on the right. Cars in the big tub, marbles in the small. Then he noticed dust on his dresser. "Ooohhh, my dresser is dusty. You need to clean that!" He made me vacuum, dust, and help sort everything. When we were just about done, he started pulling things out of his closet. I quickly said, "Jonathan, don't take those things out! We just put everything away!?!" "But," he whined, "these aren't mine!!!!! This is Matthew's" as he held up a car. "This is Zackie's," as he held up a ball, etc. He had little piles everywhere. He wants to return everything that is not his. And he said that no one is allowed in his room anymore. He needs it to stay clean. I could go on and on, but it was quite a day. He completed so many things: cleaned his room, washed his stuff, made a Christmas list, wrote a letter to Santa, made a list of people to visit and pictures to draw, and talked of all the things he still had left to do.

While we were lying in bed, waiting for Mickey and vee-vee to come out of the dryer, Jonathan said that he had a few questions. He rolled over, and in a very somber, serious tone said, "Mom, what am I going to do in heaven? The question caught me off guard. I replied that he could do anything he wanted – that there will be lots of things to do. "Where will I sleep?" I wasn't sure how to respond. I was about to say that I didn't know, when he answered his own question with, "They need to build some hotels!!" Then he asked "Where do they keep the food?" And what do I do if I have to go to the bathroom?" I told him that I didn't know, but that there were a lot of people in heaven, and that I was sure they had everything all worked out!

I am a bit shook up by all that happened today. It is obvious that he knows that he is going to die and wants to be prepared. We have never talked to him about this, and I have been struggling with how to address this for a long time. When you send your child off to kindergarten, you know he or she will be scared so you talk about what to expect to help calm his or her fears. We are so afraid of Jonathan dying that we have avoided broaching the topic with him. We have been leaving a four-year-old to fend for himself! I decided to take this opportunity to talk openly with Jonathan. So we had another long conversation. I didn't use words like 'if you die," instead I said "when you die." We talked about everything–God, Jesus, heaven, the Bible, what we know, what we don't, his disease, why things happen, what you can control, what you can't, and most importantly, about not being afraid. It was a very special conversation. We made a pact that I would not be afraid if he wasn't afraid. He said that he is not afraid and knows that Jesus will take care of him. I wonder if Jonathan was really sent here to teach us all a lesson …

Physically, Jonathan is tired and agitated. He has been sleeping a lot and complaining that his leg hurts – not as much as a few weeks ago, but still bothersome. His demeanor is more of a problem right now than his physical ailments. He is still panicked that his nose will start bleeding and wants someone to watch it for him at all times. Unfortunately, it sounds like the nosebleeds will continue to be a problem. Dr. Sawaf said the nosebleeds are a result of a low platelet count. He also said that it is conceivable that Jonathan could experience a massive hemorrhage at any time. I think the decision to transfuse again will depend on what other symptoms he might be experiencing at the time. Right now he has some energy and some things he still wants to do. It makes you really think about the words "quality of life." The problem is that we are selfish – we want him for ourselves for as long as possible. I bought an angel ornament last night. It reminded me of Jonathan. I'm still trying to determine who is really in control ...

Monday, 11/20 ~ Still moody

Well, it's 4:30 am. I have already mopped the kitchen floor, done a few loads of laundry, and spent an hour on the computer. I cannot sleep. I had a dream the other night that I went to Jonathan's funeral. Because we didn't have time to plan everything, others had done it for us, and it was all wrong. It's that control thing. So I have given up sleep.

Tom took the kids to Laura and Tim's last night as the Car-ruthers' house was on Jonathan's list of "houses to visit." Jonathan spent his time in church yesterday writing notes to each of them. He delivered them last night. Tom said that Jonathan also threw up while they were there. Because he has been so agitated, we started giving him some Ativan with his pain meds. He had a few doses of med yesterday with very little to eat. I'm guessing that's why he got sick.

We talked to the girls last night as we tucked them in. We told them that Jonathan was not doing well, and that he really could die at any time. We didn't want them to be shocked or "unprepared." We asked them if they wanted to be home with Jonathan when he died or if they would prefer to be at Grandma's or somewhere else if possible. Both of them insisted they wanted to be home with everybody around them. Elizabeth said that if Jonathan "gets sick" while she's at school, I'm supposed to come pick her up so that she can be with Jonathan. Elizabeth is openly scared and sad; Melissa is keeping her thoughts to herself. We also decided that Tom is going to take a leave of absence from work at this time. He is going to school today to set things up for a sub and plans to stay home for the next few … weeks??

Thursday, 11/23 ~ Happy Thanksgiving

I've been busy getting ready for Thanksgiving and haven't had time to update. We are hosting dinner this year for about 35 people. We have our house decorated for both Thanksgiving and Christmas as we don't want Jonathan to miss the Christmas season. The last few weeks have been an emotional roller coaster. After a bad weekend, Jonathan felt better the past few days. He played, watched cartoons, and teased Mom. Tom and I met with Pastor Jon on Tuesday and planned much of his funeral. We are getting scared. This is becoming much too real. In the past, we functioned on just "doing." Treatment and hospital visits consumed most of our time and energy. There really wasn't time to think about what was happening. But now our emotions are becoming very raw. I am becoming very sensitive to the words and actions of others. I heard through the grapevine this evening that one "friend" no longer calls because the updates are just "too hard to handle." Oh—and I'm also giving up on the anti-depressant/anti-anxiety medication.

Taking the medication causes me more anxiety than not taking it at all, and I don't have 4-6 weeks for it to take effect anyway.

Jonathan is still worried about his nose. He likes to have a box of tissues close by and is constantly sniffling. We had a blood count done yesterday as a preventative measure. (We are really trying to avoid a crisis situation over the holiday weekend. We have learned that, if at all possible, you try to avoid hospitals during holidays and long weekends!) All of his counts came back low. So, Tom and Jonathan spent the night at the hospital again last night for a red blood cell and platelet transfusion. Dr. Sawaf also thinks that Jonathan may be leaking blood somewhere in his body because his count dropped so quickly. Also Dr. Sawaf warned us that Jonathan's white cell count is very low and that he is at risk of infection. We are hoping to eek out a peaceful holiday weekend, but his condition appears very fragile. Tom and I are hoping that we can find comfort in the holiday season rather than sadness. I just want my baby. Ok, now I'm crying. See, I'm an emotional basketcase ...

Friday, 11/24 ~ Feeling fine

Believe it or not, we had a great Thanksgiving. Yesterday, we celebrated with the Dilibertis. Even with a house full of people, it was a very relaxing day. Jonathan wanted to be held a lot, but found enough energy to do crafts with the kids and even play hockey with Daddy. Today we had Thanksgiving Dinner (Round 2) with my side of the family. Jonathan seemed to be feeling even better today. He teased the family with "nah, nah, na-nah, nah's" and entertained the group with knock-knock jokes. He really seems to enjoy being surrounded by family. Laurie and I broke our holiday tradition and were not out shopping at 6:00 am this morning.

Sunday, 11/26 ~ Tired again

Life is still a roller coaster. Jonathan had another great day yesterday. We went to Grandma and Grandpa E's house as it was another on Jonathan's list of houses to visit. Plus he wanted to go to the Dollar Store with Grandma E. He bought three boxes of candy canes so that he could "give them out to all his cousins." He was peppy, happy, and had a wonderful day. Today, however, he slept most of the day. He woke up at noon and said that he was tired. He then fell back asleep. He also had a few doses of pain med today. It always seems that when he feels better he tries to do everything and then wears himself out. We then got together with the Dilibertis last night partly because Jonathan wanted to draw names for Christmas. He told me he wants to go buy his gift tomorrow if he's not too tired. I still think he's working on the closure thing. Sounds like it's also time to start thinking about another blood draw. I'm not ready to face another decision yet ...

Wednesday, 11/29 ~ In limbo

Monday and Tuesday were pretty good days. Jonathan spent most of the time watching TV or videos, playing games, and sleeping on Mom. The latest problem is that he doesn't know what to eat. The five foods he used to eat "don't sound good" anymore. Some days he doesn't eat anything; other days he eats a few bites. I can con him into drinking by saying, "That's my ice water. Don't you drink up all my water!" Then of course, teasingly, he drinks it all up and laughs! But he is starting to look very thin and pale. This morning we noticed that his left eye is also starting to turn black. His right eye, the one that was radiated, is looking

swollen again and the eyelid is completely black – like someone put on way too much black eye shadow. The bridge of
his nose also looks bruised. We have been told that neuroblastoma cells often "present" in the eye area. We also did
another blood draw today. While his platelets and white
count were still very low, his hemoglobin was just slightly
low. Dr. Sawaf recommended not doing a transfusion at
this time. He said the hemoglobin count was ok for a few
more days and that transfusing the platelets would only last
a day or two anyway. So we decided to wait a few more days.
Who knows? Maybe platelets are overrated. Jonathan was
glad to hear that we didn't have to go to the doc tonight.
Jonathan wants to see "Rugrats in Paris" with his sisters.
We are going to get the girls out of school early tomorrow
and go see the movie. His eye is getting darker …

Thursday, 11/30 ~ Pretending that everything is ok
We had another emotional conversation with Jonathan last
night. Tom, Jonathan, and I were lying in bed, and Jonathan
was particularly chatty. He then became a bit more serious
and wanted to know "why" he didn't have to go to the doc
last night. He's getting old enough to understand what's
going on and to ask real questions. Just like I want to know
and understand what's going on, I feel that he also wants
and has a right to know what is happening. So we calmly
told him that the blood test showed that he was not getting
any better and that his body was slowly dying. (For some
reason, I thought that sounded better than telling him that
the "bad cells" were taking over his body.) He immediately
started crying, not a soft or screaming cry, just a deep down,
heartfelt cry. Tom and I tried to console him by telling him
that it was going to be ok, that he needn't cry, that he
shouldn't be afraid, etc. I then looked at Tom and cried,

"This is silly!! If you told an adult they were dying, they would cry and be afraid, too. What do we expect him to do??" Then we all started crying. After a few minutes, Jonathan's crying softened, and he whimpered, "I'm just scared." We then tried explaining that even though his body was dying, that he, as a person, was not. We reminded him of all the people he knew who were already in heaven and talked about all who would join him at some later time. As we named people he knew, he stopped to add "that only those who believe in Jesus will go to heaven." Tom and I exchanged glances. I can only hope that he was comforted by his thoughts and not burdened. A few minutes later, he stopped crying. He then said in his chipper, happy voice, "You need to call Pastor Jon. I need to know everything about heaven before I go." We responded that it was too late to call Pastor Jon at the moment, but that we would call him first thing in the morning.

He then asked about Mickey and his blanket. "Will I be able to take Mickey and vee-vee with me when I go to heaven?" He then sighed and said, "No, I don't think so." So he reluctantly put us in charge of caring for his most prized belongings. And if we cannot carry out the task dutifully, Mickey and vee-vee are supposed to be passed to Melissa and Elizabeth. It was obvious that the "chain of command" was not as important as the fact that they remain deeply cherished.

Jonathan woke up in the middle of the night and told me I wasn't "snugging" him tight enough. He also reminded me that I had to call Pastor Jon in the morning. I worried that he wouldn't sleep well after our talk. He said this morning, however, that he had a "really, really good dream last night." When I asked what it was about, he said he couldn't tell me. He then added, "But you will really like it."

We went to see the movie today with Aunt Laura, cousins, Jess and Sam, and the girls. Jonathan wasn't feeling well when we left the house, but he still wanted to go. Ten minutes into the show he looked up at me with a smile and said, "This is a good movie, Mom." A few minutes later he said he felt like he was going to throw up. So he and I spent the next 15-20 minutes pacing the lobby. You could tell that he just wanted to feel better so that he could enjoy the show. We finally went back into the theater, and he slept on my lap through the rest of the movie. Melissa didn't think it was right to be missing school to go to the show. Elizabeth didn't think it was a problem.

Tom and I also made a few decisions regarding Jonathan's "final arrangements." We shared our decisions with our family and asked that they support our wishes. We are finding that these are very personal decisions. Luckily, Tom and I have agreed on most things so far. We are struggling with what to do with Mickey and vee-vee, though. Jonathan has never been without his blanket. It has been through surgery, chemo, radiation, on boats, planes, and balloons, dragged through the streets, hung from his neck—but always with him. And Mickey is his "friend." Jonathan takes him wherever he goes, shares with him his daily experiences, and snuggles him tightly when he sleeps at night. It sounds like an easy decision … but we want them.

December 2000

Friday, 12/1 ~ It's not ok
Jonathan slept in late today but woke up feeling pretty good.

Tom and I decided we wanted to set up a transfusion for sometime tonight or tomorrow. We called and left a message with Dr. Sawaf. We were then sitting on the couch watching GAS (an obnoxious TV network that Jonathan loves) while we waited for Pastor Jon to arrive per Jonathan's request. Jonathan said that he might not talk to Pastor Jon, but that we could ask him his list of questions. All of a sudden, Jonathan started screaming that his head hurt. He said that he had a "really, really, really bad" headache. We had just given him some morphine, but quickly gave him some more. We also tried some Motrin and cold compresses. He was still screaming. Of course, in the middle of this, Pastor Jon arrived, and someone wanted to sell me magazines on the phone. Jonathan, still crying uncontrollably, insisted that we all play Candy Land. We had to draw for him, move for him, etc., while he held his head, but we had to play the whole game. He just wanted to enjoy his visit with Pastor Jon. Tom finally calmed him down and lay down with him in the bedroom. Jonathan said that I needed to ask Pastor Jon his questions. After hearing the questions, Pastor Jon sat at the kitchen counter and wrote out his responses on sheets of paper. We are extremely grateful for all that Pastor Jon has done for us. Jonathan has forged a special bond with him and is very comforted by his words and presence. Later in the day, Jonathan listened carefully as we read Pastor Jon's answers to his questions. He seemed to feel a bit better, but said that he is still afraid of going to heaven.

Dr. Sawaf called back this afternoon. He again suggested that we wait a day or so before transfusing. I don't like knowing that, in making these decisions, we are partly responsible for Jonathan's comfort and well-being. But I also know that prolonging life is not always the best option. I don't think the transfusion will ever take place. Jonathan didn't eat much today and had a lot of pain meds. By evening, he was nauseated, throwing up, and said that his body hurt. By late evening, he said his back hurt, he couldn't turn over, and he couldn't stand. Feeling like things had gotten progressively worse throughout the day, I had a complete, major, emotional meltdown. I could go into details, but I really don't want to relive it. Suffice it to say that Tom didn't know what to do with me, and I ended up sitting outside on the front porch in my nightgown crying hysterically at 3:00 am with the cold winter wind blowing in my face. My frustration is not having anyone who really understands how I feel. I don't think Tom even understands how I feel. It is also even hard to talk about this with family. We don't want to talk in front of Jonathan, and I don't want to leave him, so there is no time to talk, vent, unwind, or gather opinions. I think the long cry and freezing winds helped zap me back in place. I felt better afterwards.

Jonathan spent most the night with his head hanging over a bucket feeling like he was going to throw up. In between, he was teasing me, calling me a mutt-yo head, asking me if I thought he was more pipsqueak or more fwerp (I call him a pipsqueak-twirp. He is definitely more pipsqueak!), and deciding whose turn it would be to sleep with him next. He finally fell asleep about 4:00 am. I got a few hours of sleep early this morning as the girls were gone last night. Melissa spent the night at Michelle's, and Elizabeth was at Anna's.

Saturday, 12/2 ~ Very uncomfortable

It is actually 3:30 am Sunday morning (Mom can't sleep), but we'll call it Saturday. We had another difficult day.

Jonathan is getting even worse. He has lost all of his energy and looks very frail. He is very uncomfortable and cannot move his legs or his back. He wants to be held constantly by Mom or Dad, but we are having a difficult time moving him or changing his position. He hasn't thrown up but still feels nauseated. He doesn't talk much, but when he does, it is with a very strained voice. We have been giving him both morphine and Ativan. I called hospice this morning to ask about getting a pump to begin round-the-clock pain meds. But, deep down, he is still Buzz. This morning, in his tiny voice, he said that he wanted to go to Chuck-E-Cheeses today and then to Grandma D's so that he could beat Grandpa in pool again. By midday, I convinced him that we should probably stay home today. We agreed that if he felt better tomorrow, we would go then.

Grandma D's sisters and Nicole's Mom came over last night. They all wanted to see Jonathan. We had a really nice visit and were comforted to know that they wanted to be here. I know some wonder if they should come, but we want nothing more than to be surrounded by friends and family. Jonathan, especially, seems to enjoy the company.

Right now, he is sleeping pretty soundly. He woke up a short while ago and asked for some more pain med. Before he fell back asleep, we talked a bit. He wanted to make sure that I didn't forget about Chuck-E-Cheeses and Grandpa D's. He also said that he wanted to have the "whole family" over tomorrow. I asked him if he knew how much I loved him. He said "yes" and asked, "Do you know how much I love everybody? Infinity times around the world and million thousand." It's hard to beat that!

Sunday, 12/3 ~ So hard to believe

Jonathan is not doing well at all. He spent the whole day
lying on the couch, barely able to speak or move. It is even
a struggle to understand his words at times. As pained as
he sounds, I still like to hear his voice and know what he is
thinking. I wish I could say he looks peaceful, but he looks
pitiful—just like a rag doll. But his sweet personality still
comes through. When he woke up this morning he again
said he wanted "everyone" to come over. So … we had the
whole family over. His cousins all brought him cards and
pictures. Surrounding him on the couch, they shared their
notes and artwork. He then asked his cousins if they would
bring down some of his "friends" (stuffed animals) from
his bedroom for him. As they placed the stuffed animals all
around him, he smiled and quietly said, "That makes me
soooo happy." He closed his eyes and lay on the couch as
the whole family sat around him and talked. I know that is
what he wanted. At one point, he whispered to me to play
the Tarzan song, "You'll Be in My Heart." I don't think anyone noticed, but I know he was playing the song for them.
If you listen to the words carefully, you'll see why. And
when Tom burped, Jonathan quickly opened his eyes and
said in his little, raspy voice, "You didn't say 'xcuse me',
Daddy." Jonathan perked up a bit as everyone was getting
ready to leave. He didn't want everyone to go. He made a
point of reaching up and touching each person as they left.

This afternoon, it was Melissa who had an emotional meltdown. When she gets upset and cries, she often yells out
loud and talks to herself. (It's actually very helpful. I always
make it a point to listen, so I know exactly what she's upset
about.) Through her tears I hear her say, "But it's just not
fair! I want MY Buzz. He's my little brother, and I want him

to stay here!!" Not that I'm much more emotionally prepared to deal with this myself, but I went upstairs and
hugged her, and said, "Maybe we need to get Bit and Daddy
and have a family meeting." But that didn't help. It just set
her off again. "If Buzz isn't there, then it isn't a family
meeting!" So we had a partial-family meeting—me, Melissa,
Elizabeth, and Daddy. We talked with the girls about everything—from the spiritual circle of life to the practical "what
should we do with his stuff." They asked lots of questions
and even laughed a little. Elizabeth came up with the idea
of turning his room into "The Buzz Museum." The basement will also now be called the 'Mint (Buzz's word for
basement). Later in the evening, Melissa disappeared for a
while. When she returned, she handed Grandma D a poem
she wrote about Jonathan. It was beautiful. We are getting
a large collection of things that the girls are writing and
drawing about themselves and Jonathan. As I unpack their
backpacks and look through their school work, I am reminded that these thoughts are always with them.

By the way, I've given up tracking Jonathan's pain med. We
have given him so much pain medication the past few days,
I just can't keep up. Just end it with a logarithmic curve.
Mom's intuition is that we're down to days ...

Wednesday, 12/6 ~ Platelet anxiety
I have so much to say and so little time, that I don't know
where to start. I feel like I first need to pause and publicly
acknowledge all that is going on around us. While we may
seem very self-absorbed at the moment, we are just amazed
and humbled by the outpouring of love and support that
we are receiving from others. Meals continue to show up at
our house every day. Friends and neighbors continually find

new ways to help. The girls' teachers continue to make our family news part of their daily lessons. Small gifts, cards, letters, and emails arrive daily from friends, neighbors, colleagues, students, ex-students, friends of friends, etc. Collectively, these small gestures provide great strength. It is so comforting to know that we are surrounded by such special friends and wonderful people. Thank you all very, very much!

Jonathan pretty much wants Mom and Dad at his side at all times. It's really ok because I'm afraid to leave the house anyway. He now spends most of his time lying on the couch because it is difficult to move him and, sadly, almost impossible to hold him. At times you can stroke his cheek or rub his head but, in general, he doesn't like to be touched. His voice is very quiet and often muffled. At times it is a struggle to understand what it is he wants. Today he asked for frickin nuggets (his word for chicken nuggets that's always been one of our favorites!) He sleeps about 75% of the time and is generally agitated when he is not. But in between, he still surprises us with hints of his true personality. Yesterday, when he first woke up, he said, "Mom, I have something important to tell you." I was expecting something profound, but instead he said, "If you go to internet.com on the computer and click, you can win lots of money." He then drifted off to sleep again. (In hindsight, I probably should have clicked!) Last night, after kissing Grandma E goodnight, he whispered, "Don't let the bed bugs bite." The issue of the day is that he wants someone to take him to 7-Eleven so that he can pick out his "own" candy. In trying to appease him, I think we have purchased at least one of every kind of candy. He still perks up each evening as he looks through the day's mail full of notes, cards and small gifts.

We also started Jonathan on an IV pump a few days ago. The pump is about the size of a calculator, and it dispenses pain medication around the clock. If at any time he seems to need more, we can press a button to inject an extra dose. It is designed to keep the level of morphine in his system at a constant level. Now, two days later, I don't know if this was a good idea or not. Jonathan has been complaining that the needle hurts, and he seems uptight about being "connected" to the pump. When we asked about detaching it, we found out that we can't remove it now due to his low platelet count. The nurse explained that if Jonathan starts to bleed, he does not have enough platelets to stop the bleeding. With his cracked lips, itchy nose, and pokey needle, it's just something else to cause me stress.

It has been a crazy few days. We have had a house full of people for the past three days, and in between, Tom and I have been working on a slide show and video collage for Jonathan's funeral. Immersed in happy photos and funny video clips, it is easy to deny all that is happening.

Thursday, 12/7 ~ Thank you, everyone …
Wow. I wish I could harness all the love and support that we are feeling. It is a constant reminder as to what is really important in life. We especially enjoy reading your entries in the Guestbook. Thanks for taking the time to sign. I also received an email from our internet provider today. He was shocked at the amount of traffic this site was getting and decided to check it out for himself. Perhaps more people read this than I realize.

Jonathan is still about the same. We increased his dose of morphine but haven't noticed much difference in his demeanor or comfort. He is getting increasingly frustrated at not being able to move or do anything. His diet today consisted of one frozen fish stick, three Starbursts, and lots of yellow – and only yellow – candy Runts. He wanted Taco Bell for dinner, but doesn't like tacos or anything else they serve on the menu. It's getting hard trying to keep him happy! He also just called me a Mutt-yo head. He's still a pipsqueak!

My brother, Michael, from Washington DC, drove home today. I'm glad that he came now so that he and Jonathan can see one another.

Sunday, 12/10 ~ Still hanging in there

Three days later and I'm back up and running. I have been having computer woes for some time now. Michael reformatted my computer and installed a second hard drive. It should make working and posting a little easier. Thanks, Michael!

Jonathan is still doing ok, but we are having some problems controlling his pain. When he was taking oral morphine, we could just up the dose as needed. With the pump, it is a programmed infusion rate. If we want to increase the dose, we have to call our hospice nurse, who then calls his doctor, who then writes an order, and then a hospice nurse or home care nurse has to come out and physically reprogram the pump. We increased his dose slightly last Friday morning but by evening, it was still not enough. Friday night, Jonathan woke up screaming and crying that his body hurt and that he needed more med. The pump only allows us to give him an extra dose every 15 minutes, and he was wanting more than that. Hospice came back early Saturday morning and significantly increased the dose. It was like night and day. Although he still cannot roll over or sit up by himself, he looked much more comfortable. He then asked for paper, scissors, tape, and markers so he could "make a project" for Nurse Karen, his favorite New York nurse. (Without many platelets, though, we skipped the scissors!) Later in the day, he wanted a variety of things from around the house. He was comfortable enough that Tom was able to carry him from room to room gathering his requests. From his room, he wanted his farm and farm animals. Back on the couch, we set up the farm on a table in front of him, and tried to hold him so he could play. But he ended up frustrated that he couldn't sit comfortably or move his body or the farm animals the way he wanted to. With the comfort provided by the higher dose, we were able to give him a nice sponge bath (lying on the bathroom counter) and wash his hair. He also slept well and wanted to be snuggled. We haven't been able to lie that close to him in weeks!

This morning, it was obvious that the comfort was wearing off. Perhaps yesterday was just a "good day" or maybe his pain meds need to be adjusted again. Even though he was uncomfortable, he still wanted to be held by someone most of the day. Mom, Dad, Grandma E, Aunt Laura, and Uncle Tim were the lucky recipients. Somewhere along the way, he also started charging $1 to anyone who eats at our house or holds him—except for Aunt Laura. He charged her $5. Right now, he's raking in the cash. He also collects up front. And you have to put the money in his Red Wings wallet "with the heads facing the right way."

He is soooo much like his daddy!!

Tom and I were able to sneak away for a short time today to visit the funeral home. The funeral director had ordered a few caskets for us to see. They were nice, if you can say that, and we choose a light oak one with satin lining. They are going to replace the light blue satin with light blue velvet. Jonathan likes his blankets to be soft, not shiny.

The highlight of our weekend was a surprise visit from Santa Claus! Santa came while the whole family was here last night and had presents for all of the cousins. Jonathan then read Santa his whole Christmas list (a bunch of toys he saw on TV), but said that he most wants a new scooter for Christmas this year. It breaks my heart to know that he hasn't given up riding his scooter down the street. When Santa asked Melissa what she wanted for Christmas, she whispered to Santa that her brother has cancer and that, for her present, she just wants him to get better. Her wish made Santa melt, too. The kids were thrilled that Santa just happened to choose our house for a visit, and we were glad that we happened to have a lot of cameras close by.

Hospice is coming out soon to increase Jonathan's pain med again. We are expecting snow and blizzard-like conditions this evening. We don't want to get snowed in and need an increase tomorrow!

Tuesday, 12/12 ~ Buried in snow
The hospice nurse came yesterday in the middle of the huge snowstorm. I really don't know how she got through, but we are extremely, extremely, grateful for her effort. Although the falling snow was beautiful, I did worry about

having a medical emergency in the middle of a blizzard. They have already called school off for both today and tomorrow. There is always something magical about a "snow day" – especially for teachers!

I think we have Jonathan's pain under control. He slept most of the day yesterday, but when he was awake, he was very alert. We were also able to give him a bath again. He is looking much paler, and he was already pale weeks ago. Last night, we watched the video from Santa's visit two days ago. He looked so "sickly" in the video. I guess we just don't see it day to day. We still see him as Buzz – just like always. When I hold him and snuggle him, everything seems just like normal. Today we watched more cartoons, and he even drew the Blue's Clues in his handy, dandy notebook! I told the hospice nurse yesterday that I couldn't believe that he has come this far without any blood transfusions. She said that she was surprised too. I truly feel like we're in a "holding pattern." I treasure every minute I have with him but feel guilty that I am "waiting" for it all to end. I will not leave the house, because I cannot bear to not be here when it eventually does. I am staying up most nights – like all night – re-energizing with the peace and solitude. I get my catnaps while holding Jonathan off and on throughout the day. Melissa and Elizabeth's classes are holding a Bake Sale this week with all of the proceeds going to cancer research. The girls are having to grow up much too quickly …

Wednesday, 12/13 ~ Still buried in snow
It has been a pretty peaceful day. The snow is keeping everyone away. (Well Grandma and Grandpa E, Uncle Sal and Anna, and Uncle Dan and Aunt Nic all made it through!) Jonathan also said that angels came to get him

last night. When I asked what happened, he said he told them that he didn't want to go with them, that he "wanted to stay with Momma and Daddy." I personally like the thought that there were angels in our bedroom!

We have also had to temper our ways with Jonathan. In the past, we have run to countless stores (McDonald's, Target, Toys R Us, Wendy's, Kroger, the Dollar Store, etc.), many times more than once in the same day, because he needed something. Usually, by the time we returned, he was sleeping or it was no longer an issue. With the snow still falling, we are perfecting the great art of distraction. When he asked to go to 7-Eleven, we asked if he wanted to watch some cartoons. When he told me to hurry up and get him dressed because Uncle Chris was coming over to pick him up (I don't know where he thought they were going!), I countered with, "Would you like a fish stick?" He forgot all about Uncle Chris. The highlight of the day was the bathroom excursion. I was getting ready to mop the bathroom floor and had just removed all of the rugs. Next thing I know, Tom is behind me carrying Jonathan saying, "Uhhh … he wants to go potty in the big potty!"—both of us knowing that this was going to be a disaster. The problem is that he cannot sit, stand, point, or aim. Before we knew it, he was peeing all over the bathroom—two whole days worth!! Jonathan was then upset about the mess and that he got some on Daddy (that part made Mom smile!). One bath later, everyone was fresh and clean!! It's good to know that the kidneys are still functioning.

Hospice came by this again morning and upped his pain meds. He complained off and on last night that his legs were hurting. They also inserted an extra section of IV tubing that will allow us to give his Ativan and any other meds through the tube rather than orally. It's nice to know we have easy access to provide medication in case of an emergency.

In between caring for Jonathan, Tom and I have been working on the funeral slide show and video montage. After many suggestions, we decided on four songs for the video collage: "When I Look into Your Eyes" by Firehouse, "I Could Not Ask for More" by Edwin McCain, "Allstar" by Smashmouth, and "Can You Feel the Love Tonight" by Elton John. We saved Jonathan's favorite song, "You'll Be in My Heart," from Tarzan, for the final slide show. Also, while looking for songs for the video, I stumbled upon another song called Power of Your Love by Hillsongs. Tom and I agreed that it would be the perfect song to end the service. Things are slowly coming together …

Thursday, 12/14 ~ Third snow day: Mom's losing it

The kids were home from school again today! I cannot ever remember having three snow days in a row!! Today, I felt like a mom who wanted the kids back in school. Tom was out running errands, and I was immobile on the couch holding Jonathan. The girls, like all bored kids, were driving me crazy with all of their simple requests. "Mom, I'm bored. What can I do? Mom, can you drive me to so-and-so's house? Mom, can so-and-so spend the night?" Agghh! I wanted to just yell, "Can't you see that I need to be with Jonathan right now and that after he dies we can do all of those things!!" Of course I didn't … I tried to be a good Mom. I told them that now was not a good time, but that we could do so in a few weeks.

Then I had a guilt episode. In all of the snow play, the zipper on Melissa's winter coat broke yesterday and is not fixable. So I needed to get her to the mall to get a new winter coat before she heads back to school – one good thing about the extra snow day. But because I didn't want to leave the house, I asked my sister, Laurie, if she would take Melissa out to get a new coat this evening. Melissa usually likes shopping with Aunt Laurie but this time asked, "Why can't you take me to the mall?" I told her that I couldn't because I needed to stay home with Jonathan. I then spent the afternoon holding Jonathan while the girls played together on the computer. As I held Jonathan, I thought about what this situation must look like to the girls. Mom and Dad, and everyone else, do anything and everything for Jonathan and then help with the girls when, or if, they get a chance. I really wanted to take Melissa to the mall, partly to spend some time with her, but knew that I had to justify doing so to myself before I could go. I told myself that I have done everything that I could possibly do for Jonathan, but that I had three children who all needed me. So I told Jonathan I needed to take the girls to the mall (he said he wanted to go too, but then agreed to stay home with Daddy instead), and that I would be home soon. I was secretly letting him know that if he had any control over the situation to "wait" until Mom got home. So I left tightly holding Tom's pager and an emergency cell phone. I stopped to pick up Laurie, and we headed to the mall. Disaster always being predictable in my life, Tom paged me halfway there. First, I couldn't figure out how to use the pager, then we discovered that the "emergency" cell phone was dead, and then we chose a pay phone that rejected our calling card and many, many quarters. My heart was at my feet. We finally made it through, and Tom passed along a relevant but not "urgent, life-threatening" message. He apologized for paging me, knowing it would send me into a panic but didn't know what else to do. We agreed that any future, truly "urgent" pages would be followed by our "secret code."

Fast-forward to the mall. I discovered that I'm not as "well" as I thought I was. When the pleasant cashier said, "So, how are you today?" I wanted to punch her. I swore at the slow, meandering, Christmas shoppers in front of me who didn't "know" that I was in a hurry. And then I picked a fight with another cashier who didn't know the price of the matching mittens I was trying to buy. I tried to be "normal" but couldn't. Even Laurie noticed. She said that she will have to shop for me until I am "better." We had pizza with the Ferraris, and Grandma and Grandpa D stopped by for dessert.

Jonathan was really out of it today. He slept most all day and was very groggy. When he woke up and tried to say something, he sounded winded, and usually fell back asleep before completing his sentence. We gave him his first dose of Ativan in his line this morning. The hospice nurse said that it is much more potent when taken this way. I don't know if the change in his demeanor is the result of the Ativan or just another change in status, but right now, he's sleeping peacefully on Daddy. I'm almost done with the video …

Friday, 12/15 ~ Just holding on …

10:30 am, Friday morning
Jonathan slipped into a coma-like state sometime this morn-

ing. Tom and I are sitting on the couch together, taking turns holding him. We are not taking any phone calls at the moment. Please leave a message if you'd like. We'll keep you posted ...

10:30 pm, Friday night
It has been a long day. Tom and I noticed last night that Jonathan's breathing was becoming very irregular and that something had "changed." Instead of staying up all night to watch over him, we decided to go to bed with Jonathan lying between us. Although he did not respond, we talked to him, told him how much we loved him, cried a lot, and told him that is was ok to "go," and that we would be ok. This morning when we picked him up, his whole body was limp. We tried to wake him but couldn't. His heart was beating really hard and his pulse was very fast. The girls were at school, and Tom and I just wanted this time alone with him. (That's when I posted the above message.) We held him off and on but, at times, he was tossing and turning his body so much that we had to put him down. We gave him a couple of doses of Ativan and that seemed to help. I don't know if it was pain or just restlessness.

Soon after we called our families and asked everyone to spend the evening with us. Tom and I are torn between wanting to be surrounded by family when the time comes and wanting to be alone with Jonathan. I guess neither of us knows quite what to expect and how we are going to respond. Not much has changed throughout the day. Although his legs and feet appear swollen, he seems to be losing a lot of fluid. We went through a lot of Pull-Ups today! He also had a couple of bowel movements today – not too exciting to talk about unless you haven't had one in weeks! We watched a home video of Jonathan's balloon ride in October and cannot believe how vibrant he looked just two months ago. Now that the "real" end is fast approaching, my hidden emotions are starting to show. I received an email today from another mom who has been a tremendous source of strength and knowledge. Her son Robby also lost his battle to neuroblastoma. Her last sentence was of great comfort to me. "Robby will have a new friend. I've already told him to look for Jonathan." I don't want him to be alone …

2:50 am Saturday, 12/16 ~ Jonathan joined Jesus
I just wanted everyone to know … I will post again later. Even though we knew this was coming, it is just so hard to believe. I am just … numb.

Saturday, 12/16 ~ Summary of Friday night and Saturday
Tom was half-sleeping on the couch with Jonathan stretched across him. Jonathan was still unresponsive and the depth and sound of his breathing changed each time he moved his head. I think both Tom and I knew that the end was very, very near. I think I knew that there was going to be a lot of activity at our house in the coming days, so I did some quick housecleaning. I finished cleaning about 1:00 am and then decided to put the finishing touches on the funeral video. With Tom and Jonathan sleeping in the great room, I clicked away on the video at the dining room table. We really wanted the video done before Jonathan died so we knew that we would be "ready" for the funeral. I finished editing the video at 2:40 am. I then woke Tom up, told him that the video was done, and said that I was ready for bed. We then oscillated between sleeping with Jonathan on the couch or putting him in bed between us like we did

last night. We decided that he would be more comfortable sleeping between us rather than on us. I helped Tom carry him from the couch to the bedroom. When Tom picked him up, his arms and legs just fell. He was sooo limp. As we were carrying him, we again talked to him, told him that it was ok to go, and said that God and Jesus would take very good care of him. Tom then laid him gently on our bed. He kind of gasped, and we knew that this was the end. Tom was gently stroking his head, telling him that we would miss him, but that we would be ok. I looked away because I didn't want to "watch" him die. I just couldn't. He took three more similar breaths, and then … stopped. It was 2:50 am. When I turned and looked at his lifeless body lying on the bed, it was immediately obvious to me that what remained of Jonathan was just his shell. Our Buzz, the one so full of life and energy, must truly be someplace else. Then I realized that he was forever gone. And the tears just started to flow. I have never cried so hard and so deep in my life. All the while, Tom was equally immersed in his own deep sobs. We clung to one another. As open as we have been and as much as we have chosen to be surrounded by family and friends, Tom and I were both glad that we were alone with him during this time. We soon woke up Melissa and called for Elizabeth, who was attending a friend's birthday sleepover. Within minutes, Elizabeth was home, and we all gathered on the bed. We laid with Buzz and tried to share some quality time. The girls seemed to understand the permanence of the situation, but it was obvious from their questions that they had little concept of what happens next.

About 3:30 am, we called our parents and asked them to help spread the word. I then called the hospice nurse and the Funeral Director as we were directed to do. (Sometime

during this first half hour, I also posted the above few
sentences.) We asked the Funeral Director to come about
5:00 am—late enough to give us some more time yet early
enough to beat the new day. Our family started to arrive
within minutes. The girls were awake for a short time but
soon fell asleep on the couch. Tom spent much of his time
in the bedroom lying with Jonathan. I divided my time
between Jonathan and the many guests now gathered in our
home. I was also overwhelmed by the thought that this was
going to be a really long day after a night of no sleep. When
it was time, Tom carried Jonathan out to the waiting car.
Even with the room full of people, the house felt empty.

By about 8:00 am, everyone had left. With the girls still
sleeping, both Tom and I quickly fell asleep. When the girls
woke us up a few hours later, we discovered that they had
each already made a few phone calls of their own. I wish
Tom and I hadn't fallen asleep. I am sure that the girls
needed us during this time. I noticed later that Melissa had
changed the screen saver on her computer to say, "Buzz—
I really, really, (lots more really's!) love you!!!!!!!!!!!!!!!!!!!!!!!" and
Elizabeth wrote, "I love you, Buzz!" on my notepad in the
office. Melissa then wanted to go out for breakfast and
Elizabeth wanted to go back to the birthday party which
had now moved on to the skating rink. Somehow I think
that choosing to do "normal" things helped the girls escape
the pain and disbelief they were experiencing. I just wanted
to sleep. As we were preparing to leave, Pastor Jon came
by. We talked briefly with Pastor Jon, dropped Elizabeth
off at the skating rink, went out to breakfast, dropped
Melissa off back home with Grandma E, and then headed
to the funeral home for a 1:00 pm appointment. We spent
three hours finalizing details and learning about mortuary

science. By the time we got back home, Tom and I were both physically and emotionally exhausted. We spent the rest of the day surrounded by family.

Funeral Arrangements

We invite you to join us as we celebrate Jonathan's life and say our final goodbyes. Visitations will take place Tuesday and Wednesday at the Wujek-Calcaterra Funeral Home. The funeral will be Thursday at 10:00 am at Shepherd's Gate Lutheran Church, followed by a committal service at Resurrection Cemetery. Immediately after, we invite all to join us for a memorial luncheon at Fern Hill Country Club.

A Week Later

Saturday, 12/23 ~ Summary of past week

I really don't know what to say or where to start. This past week has been unbelievable and almost unbearable. Unbelievable in that so much has happened; almost unbearable in that our Buzz is gone.

Jonathan's funeral was our one last chance to do something special for him, and we wanted it to be perfect. Most importantly, we wanted the video collage and slide show to run smoothly. As a result, Tom spent a lot of time at church ironing out glitches, ensuring that each of the programs would run as expected on the church's computer system. In between, we also designed and printed our own prayer cards and funeral programs. We gathered stuffed animals and toys for the funeral home, shopped for new dresses and shoes for the girls, selected music, and tended to many other last minute details. Everyone helped pull things together.

Laura and Tim printed and folded the funeral programs. Laurie ordered flowers and had Jonathan's portraits matted so that they could be signed by guests at the visitation. Tim and Tom put together photo boards, Chris searched for music CD's, friends from school searched for easels, our parents organized the family buffets, Michael played tech support, and friends and neighbors helped with the girls. I also want to publicly say that our church, Shepherd's Gate, did so much for us. Their media crew helped ready our technology show, they picked up and installed a second video projector for the funeral service, the church band searched for and learned to play the closing song we requested, and many, many others helped behind the scenes with parking, coordination, food, and miscellaneous details. Thank you everyone for everything!! We didn't really think or feel. Even after trying to be "ready," there was still so much to do.

In the midst of all of our preparations, Elizabeth informed us that she would be unable to attend Jonathan's funeral because it was the same day and time as her first grade school play, "How the Grinch Stole Christmas." And she was Who #7 – complete with a speaking line! After hearing the date of Jonathan's funeral, however, her teacher changed the date of the performance to avoid any conflicts. We know this change affected a lot of people, and appreciate everyone's willingness to accommodate our situation.

Days prior, thinking about seeing and greeting everyone at the funeral home made me nervous. In fact, funeral homes in general make me nervous. But after visiting two or three times, and having had the grand tour – through the casket room, the visitation rooms, the garage, the employee kitchen, and asking a number of forensic science questions, we were much more at ease. Tim, Laura, and Tom took the girls and all of the cousins to the funeral home the night before the visitation so that they would know what to expect.

Tuesday, 12/19 ~ Funeral Visitation Day 1

We got to the funeral home early to finish some last minute details. We opted for an open casket but Jonathan barely looked like himself to me. In some sense, this helped me. I was again reminded that my Buzz was somewhere else, full of life. His shell didn't seem to "fit" without him in it. Tom was much more connected to Jonathan's body. To him, it was still a part of Jonathan and something that he wanted to care for and nurture until the very end. He continued to talk to Jonathan and stroke his cheek. We spent the rest of our private hour arranging things, decorating the casket (the kids covered it in stickers!), looking at the flowers, and decorating a Christmas tree with Buzz's favorite little toys and candies.

The whole afternoon and evening quickly became a blur. It was comforting to see so many people from all walks of our life. Some people said they were surprised by our "normal" demeanor; others confided that it helped them relax. I was determined to remain composed during the visitation because I was afraid that if I started crying, I might never stop. We must have been functioning on autopilot, though, because I have few recollections of the day.

Wednesday, 12/20 ~ Funeral Visitation Day 2

Again, it was nice to see so many people. While the day passed quickly, a few moments stand out in my memory.

The most heartening visit today was with another mom whose son, Michael, is also battling neuroblastoma. We met at Memorial Sloan Kettering in New York, but she is from Wisconsin. She and her family drove from Wisconsin to attend the visitation and funeral. I started crying as soon as I saw her walk in – partly because I didn't want her to think that it always ends this way.

Melissa and Elizabeth's teachers also arranged for all of their classmates (and their parents) to meet at the funeral home at 4:00 pm. We were unaware of the plan and thus very touched as we watched the girls' teachers lead their classmates into the room, each carrying a single white rose with a note attached, to give to the girls. Melissa and Elizabeth so appreciated being surrounded by their friends. And it was nice that their classmates, who had questions of their own, were able to participate in some small way. Their teachers visited for awhile and then took the girls out for dinner. Later in the evening, Uncle Dick (Tom's uncle and godfather), shared a piece of prose he had written about Jonathan's faith, and Grandpa D read a beautiful letter written by Grandma D. The final highlight of the day was Elizabeth, still standing up for her brother. While looking at the casket, one of her friends said, "He looks kind of creepy." Elizabeth quickly shot back, "He's not creepy!! He's my brother!!"

After everyone left, we lingered with our extended family. We talked with one another, and we talked to Jonathan. We slowly removed the stuffed animals and toys from his casket and left him to sleep with just Mickey and vee-vee. We gathered our things and finalized what would be taken to church. As all of this was going on, Tom just sat in a chair and cried. He was just not ready to leave his little boy. We said goodbye to Jonathan, and Pastor Jon led us in prayer. We walked out feeling very, very sad and very, very empty. We went to Laurie's for a late-night dinner and stayed for a while to visit with out-of-town relatives. When we got home, we tucked the girls in, and Tom and I talked about how surreal this whole week has been. We are still not ready to face reality.

Thursday, 12/21 ~ Jonathan's Funeral

Surprisingly, I was somewhat relaxed this morning, but the reality was setting in. Soon the casket would be closed, and I would never again be able to see Jonathan. Tom and I each found a few private moments to spend with him before others started to arrive. I was sadder now than I have ever been, but I did not want to start crying. We had put so much time into planning the funeral service, I wanted to be coherent enough to see it all come together. I found a quiet moment to kiss Jonathan and tell him goodbye for the very last time. As it neared 10:00 am and the service was about to begin, I picked up Mickey and snuggled him as I walked away from the casket. Tom spent a lot of time with Jonathan this morning. He kissed him, talked to him, and at times, just sat staring at him. He said all along that he wanted to "tuck Jonathan in one last time." I knew that I could not participate in the closing of the casket. As the song, "Somewhere, Somehow," by Michael Smith and Amy Grant played, Tom carefully removed vee-vee from Jonathan's arms and placed it over his shoulder. He then kissed Jonathan's forehead, and with the help of the funeral director, gently closed the lid of the casket. He then placed Jonathan's two stuffed angel bears amongst the flowers at one end of the casket and draped Jonathan's Red Wing's

jersey over the other. Tom looked as if his heart was melt-
ing, but he was able to carry out this final task, and for that,
he will always be Daddy. The service was everything we
wanted. Pastor Jon did a wonderful job describing Jonathan
and sharing his faith, the church band played our favorite
songs (ok, we picked them), and the girls and their cousins
all wore monogrammed Red Wings jerseys which the
owner of DC Sports at Lakeside Mall rushed to complete.
The video and slide show went off without a hitch, and
the service ended with our new favorite song, "The Power
of Your Love" by Hillsong, sung by my sister, Laurie, along
with the church band.

After the church service, many joined us at the cemetery
for the brief committal service. I am sure that most who
attended were unaware of our final plans as we had kept
our final arrangements to ourselves. Tom and I struggled
with the choice of burial or cremation. Truthfully, we were
not comfortable with either one. Early on we both assumed
that we would bury Jonathan, but then I started having
second thoughts. I didn't know how I could sleep at night
when I could picture him, a child who spent most nights
sleeping between Mom and Dad, buried in the deep, dark,
cold ground. So, we chose to have him cremated instead.
That is equally discerning, but to me, it is the lesser of two
evils. I keep focusing on the shell thing and know that he is
somewhere else feeling better than ever. This is also why
we chose to keep Mickey and vee-vee. Jonathan entrusted
us to take care of them. We didn't think that burying them
in the ground or cremating them would have been
Jonathan's definition of caring for them.

The afternoon ended with a buffet luncheon across the

street from the cemetery at Fern Hill Country Club. The angel sugar cookies iced with Jonathan's name were a thoughtful surprise. (Thank you, Janice and Mary.) We are so glad that so many of you were able to share in our final goodbye.

This will be my final entry in the Journal. I cannot believe that my Buzz is gone ...

PART FIVE

Jonathan's Gift

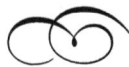

"The true measure of a life is not its length
but the fullness with which it is lived."

Ten Years Later

*I*t has taken me a long time to put our journey into words. After working on this book project for a few weeks each summer for many summers in a row, I can now see the effects of time. The days, weeks, and months following Jonathan's death were just … empty. There were many times that I tried to journal again, with the hope of sharing the aftermath with others as well, but the words just wouldn't come. I would sit in front of my computer and just sit, stare, or cry. I had few thoughts, little energy, and no motivation. I remember sleeping until noon, dragging myself out of bed, and then doing nothing the rest of the day. Luckily, I still had to be Mom. That gave me a reason for being.

Within a few weeks, the emptiness filled with emotion. I was sad, lonely, moody, grouchy, cranky, snippy, petty, and anything else "bad" you can think of. I was totally consumed with thoughts of Jonathan. Sleeping became an escape from the emotional pain I was feeling. But as soon as I woke up, I would … remember. And our house, which was always chaotic, was now uncomfortably quiet. The girls

walked and played quietly, whereas Jonathan would have
been running and chattering loudly. To fill my void, I
watched the video collage that we made for Jonathan's
funeral at least once or twice (ok, sometimes more) every
day. Yes, I was clearly depressed.

While Tom and the girls seemed a bit more stable, they
had their issues too. Melissa drew pictures of angels and
kept close tabs on Jonathan's things. With his daily antics
still fresh in our minds, she was always the first to say,
"What would Buzz be doing now?" Elizabeth carried
Jonathan's stuffed angel bears around and constantly talked
about missing her brother. While Melissa preferred to keep
her thoughts and emotions to herself, Elizabeth talked to
anybody and everybody about her brother, Buzz. Tom went
back to work right away, while I remained off for a few
more weeks. He started working out excessively and enjoyed getting together with his buddies playing cards,
playing basketball, doing anything to help him forget. He
said being with others doing normal things made him feel
better. Being with others who wanted to talk about Buzz is
all that I wanted to do.

Ironically, as the months wore on and people assumed
that we were "getting better," things actually got worse. I
felt almost dumbfounded that life could go on when
Jonathan was no longer here. And little things would just
set me off. Chatting with a new acquaintance, "So, how
many children do you have?" or an old friend, "So, how
have you been?" My mind would start racing and I would
feel an overwhelming surge of anxiety. I made a CD of the
songs we chose for Jonathan's funeral and popped it in
every morning on my drive to work. Within minutes, the
familiar tears would start to flow. It became a daily ritual,
like something I had to go through before I could start my

day. I actually preferred the distractions of work. At home, I was surrounded by the constant reminders. I didn't know what to do with his things and couldn't bear to think about it. Tom also started feeling tense and anxious. He said he just couldn't relax and was not himself. I also worried about the girls. Melissa was keeping everything inside, and Elizabeth started writing Jonathan's name instead of her own on the top of all of her school papers. I also sensed that people around us tried to avoid mentioning Jonathan thinking it might "remind" us of the situation. Did they really think that we forgot?!?

I guess it's true what they say. Time heals all wounds. Many, many months later, the fog began to lift. We purchased a curio cabinet to house some of Jonathan's most precious things: his Handy Dandy notebook, Happy Meal toys, Red Wings puck, Yankees baseball, WWJD bracelet, Grover beanie baby, Mickey Mouse hat, etc. We framed his Red Wings jersey and packed away most of his things. (I'm not sure I'll ever be ready to get rid of them!) A few years later, I could even share Jonathan's story with others with minimal tears. Jonathan's bedroom became our upstairs TV room, but it still looked like Jonathan's room. One Christmas, Liz asked to move into his bedroom: not to just move in, but to make his room her own. So after one last look, a deep breath, and memories of the past, we painted Jonathan's navy blue walls a bright shade of pink.

Over the years, I have also come to know and take comfort in what I call "Buzzisms." Buzzisms are those little "coincidental" things that happen at just the right time that make you realize the world extends beyond our earthly presence. My favorite was the day, months after Jonathan died, when Melissa was crying uncontrollably in the middle of Target saying that she didn't want to go on a family vacation without Buzz. Within moments, "You'll Be in My Heat" started playing over the Target loudspeaker. On the same trip, the girls received Mickey Mouses as their Happy Meal toys, and we walked into a Wendy's covered in posters with the tagline "It's all the Buzz." Over the years I've experienced enough Buzzisms to believe that they really exist – if you are a willing recipient.

After years of witnessing and receiving acts of kindness from others, Tom and I felt the need to "give back" in some way. We originally established a childhood cancer support organization in Jonathan's name, but soon realized that we could do even greater good if we combined our efforts with others trying to do the same. Together with some friends, family, and health professionals from St. John Hospital, we founded Candlelighters Childhood Cancer Foundation of Michigan, a local chapter of a national, non-profit organization. The organization strives to support, educate, and advocate for children who have, or have had cancer and their families. The organization recently changed its name to the Michigan Childhood Cancer Foundation, or MCCF for short. Helping others in this capacity has been a big part of our healing process.

Melissa and Elizabeth are now both young adults. The effects of losing their brother at such a young age show up in bits and pieces of their respective personalities. They are both well-adjusted, bright, caring, and compassionate individuals. Melissa possesses a deep sense of realism and responsibility, yet is happily balanced by an engaging, down-to-earth personality. Elizabeth is a bit softer, preferring to lead and assist others in a more simple manner, often behind the scenes. While they lost part of their childhood innocence, they gained a meaningful appreciation of one another. Unlike many siblings, the girls share more best-friend characteristics than sibling rivalries.

Jonathan continues to be a constant presence in our lives as we exchange Buzz jokes and include him often in our daily discussions. Tom eventually left education and took a new job that involves a lot of travel. I continue to teach. We are changed, but we have once again found peace and happiness.

As the years passed, our extended family also continued to grow. Nephew Christopher was born to Lynn and Sal, ten years after Anna. Dan and Nicole had two children – Cole Daniel and Luke Jonathan, about the same time. A few years later, my brother, Michael, married Becky and their son, William Matheson, was born a year later. While the new cousins are still young, we have gone out of our way to share a bit of Buzz with all of them. From Toy Story books to monogrammed jerseys, I can only hope that they grow to find a connection to Jonathan in some way. I am certain that Jonathan looks after them all.

Reflecting now, I also have a much bigger, broader, realistic picture of Jonathan's medical condition and treatment. He had a lot of odds stacked against him. Would the outcome be the same if Jonathan were diagnosed today? Yes, I think so. Unfortunately, medical researchers have made little strides in treating high-risk neuroblastoma. While we were hoping for a cure with the monoclonal antibodies, a review of the current literature reveals that the antibody treatments are still in a state of relative infancy. We are glad that Jonathan was able to contribute to this growing body of research in some small way. And we are most inspired by and indebted to the folks who make searching for medical cures part of their daily job. Hopefully, the day will come when all who are affected by this deadly disease can rejoice.

Lastly, we have no regrets. Both Tom and I know that we left no stoned unturned and always acted with Jonathan's best interests in mind. As his earthly time came to a close, we are grateful that we had the time and opportunity to say goodbye. Jonathan reminded us to find joy in each new day and that true peace and acceptance comes from within. Most importantly, Jonathan taught us that the world is a much bigger place than we know and understand. I know where he sleeps.

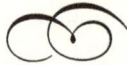

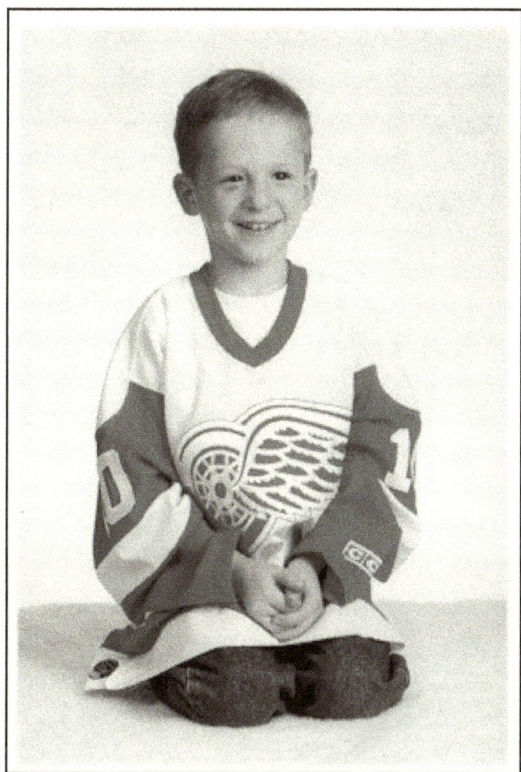

JONOTHON

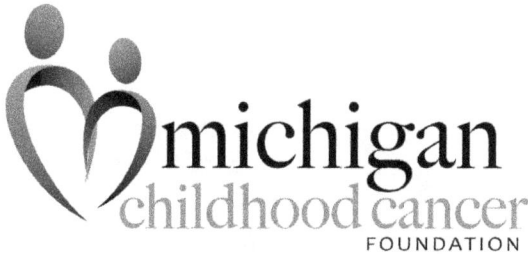

Michigan Childhood Cancer Foundation

The Michigan Childhood Cancer Foundation (MCCF) is a recognized 501(c)3 non-profit organization dedicated to serving childhood cancer families in Michigan. The foundation aims to support, educate, and advocate for children who have, or have had cancer, and their families by offering support programs, educational resources, and participating in advocacy events.

For more information about how MCCF can help or how you can get involved, please visit our website at www.miccf.org. We are always looking for new volunteers and/or new ways to expand our partnerships.

"Because kids can't fight cancer alone."

www.ingramcontent.com/pod-product-compliance
Lightning Source LLC
Chambersburg PA
CBHW031300310326
41914CB00116B/1682/J